AI for Veterinarians

A Practical Guide to AI Tools, Clinical Documentation, and Workflows for the Modern Veterinary Practice

Arrow Jay Publishing
Fort Pierce, Florida | 2026

A Note on AI-Assisted Writing:
This book was researched, structured, and written with the assistance of AI tools. All content has been reviewed, edited, and approved by the publisher. The use of AI in the preparation of this manuscript is consistent with the principles described throughout this book, that AI is a productivity tool that amplifies human judgment, not a replacement for it.

AI for Veterinarians is part of the AI for Professionals Series.

ISBN (Paperback): 978-1-964326-08-5

ISBN (eBook): 978-1-964326-09-2

First Edition, 2026

Contents

Introduction

Let's be honest with each other right from the start.

You didn't spend four years of undergraduate coursework, four years grinding away at veterinary school, and somewhere between $150,000 and $250,000 in student loans so you could spend your evenings in a parking lot finishing charts on your phone. You didn't go through gross anatomy, clinical rotations, and boards so that your most consistent daily experience would be staring at a blinking cursor trying to remember exactly how you worded the discharge instructions for Mrs. Henderson's post-op Cocker Spaniel.

But here you are. And if you're like most of the veterinarians practicing right now, the paperwork isn't a minor inconvenience. It is a genuine weight. It follows you home. It keeps you at the clinic an hour past when your last patient left. It sits in the back of your mind on your days off, a low hum of things undone and notes unfinished.

A 2025 Federation of Veterinarians of Europe report found that 64% of veterinarians said their administrative workload had doubled in recent years, with another 29% reporting a slight increase. The single most time-consuming task? Prescribing and dispensing documentation, with many veterinarians spending up to ten hours a week on it alone. Most respondents also reported that more than half of their administrative work is unpaid. Burnout research from the AVMA, Merck Animal Health, and others consistently identifies administrative burden as a meaningful contributor to the stress veterinary professionals carry home with them.

Ten hours a week. That is a day and a quarter of your working life, every single week, spent not practicing medicine.

This book exists because there is a tool that can cut a meaningful chunk of that time. Not eliminate it. Medicine requires human judgment and human accountability, and this book will be very clear about where those lines are. But cut it? Yes. Significantly. Veterinarians and other healthcare professionals using AI documentation tools report reductions in documentation time anywhere from 40% to 75%, depending on how they use them and how complex their cases run.

That is hours back. Real hours. Hours you can spend with patients, with clients, with your family, or just with enough quiet in your head to remember why you chose this work in the first place.

Here is how this book is structured, and why it is structured this way.

Chapter 1 comes before everything else because it covers the ethics, the limits, and the professional obligations you need to understand before you pick up any new tool. That is not a legal disclaimer dressed up as a chapter. It is genuinely the most important thing in the book. If you understand where the guardrails are before you start, everything you learn afterward lands in the right context. You will use these tools with more confidence, fewer second-guesses, and a clear sense of what you are and are not doing.

After that, this book gets practical. Chapter 2 maps your full documentation universe, because most veterinarians have never actually counted how many distinct document types they produce in a week, and the number is usually a surprise. Chapters 3 through 9 are hands-on, specific, and built around the actual workflows of a working veterinary practice. Chapter 11 is a prompt library you can flip to during your actual workday and copy directly. Chapter 12 is a 30-day plan if you want a guided path from "never used AI" to "AI is part of my daily workflow."

You do not have to read this straight through. If you're already sold on the concept and just want to get started, Chapter 3 will get you going. If you're skeptical about the ethics, Chapter 1 will either settle those concerns or tell you exactly what you need to think about more carefully. If you're a practice owner trying to figure out the operational side, Chapter 7 is yours.

One thing this book will never do is oversell. AI tools are genuinely useful. They're also genuinely limited. They make mistakes with confidence. They can produce output that sounds authoritative and is factually wrong. They do not know your patients, your clients, your state's regulations, or your own clinical judgment, and they never will. Everything in this book is built around that reality, not around hype.

You became a veterinarian to take care of animals. This book is about getting the paperwork out of the way so you can do that better.

Let's get to work.

Chapter 1

The Rules of the Road - AI Ethics, Limits, and Your License

Before we talk about what AI can do for your practice, we need to talk about what it cannot do, what it should never do, and where your professional responsibility sits in all of this. Not because this is the cautious chapter you have to get through before the useful stuff starts, but because understanding the limits is what makes everything else safe to use.

Think of it this way. A brand-new associate vet on their first week can observe surgery, can ask questions, and can help prep a patient. What they cannot do is pick up a scalpel and make the first incision without supervision. Not because they're incompetent. They may be brilliant. But the professional and legal structure of veterinary medicine requires that certain decisions and actions be made by the licensed practitioner who holds responsibility for the patient. AI is something like that new associate, except it never gets licensed, it never develops actual judgment, and it isn't aware that it's making mistakes when it makes them.

Once you've got that mental model, the rest of this chapter is just filling in the specifics.

What AI Actually Is - And Why That Matters Clinically

The AI tools we are talking about in this book, ChatGPT, Claude, Gemini, and similar large language models, are text prediction systems. They were trained on enormous amounts of text from the internet, books, articles, and other sources, and they learned to predict what words are likely to follow other words. When you ask one of these tools to draft a discharge instruction, it is not looking up the correct answer. It is generating text that matches the pattern of what a discharge instruction typically looks like, based on what it saw in training.

That distinction matters enormously in a clinical context.

A well-written discharge instruction and a wrong discharge instruction can look identical coming out of an AI tool. The language is fluent. The format is correct. The confident tone gives nothing away. The error, if there's one, might be a drug interaction that was not flagged, a dosage that is close but not quite right for the patient's weight, or a contraindication that applies to this species but not the species the training data was weighted toward.

This phenomenon has a name in the industry: hallucination. AI tools produce incorrect information with the same fluency and apparent confidence as correct information. They do not know the difference. They cannot flag their own errors. And in veterinary medicine, an error that makes it into a patient record or a client handout without being caught is a liability event, and more importantly, a harm to an animal.

The rule that flows from this is simple and non-negotiable: every single AI output that touches patient care must be reviewed by you before it becomes part of a record or goes home with a client. Every time. No exceptions. We will repeat this throughout the book because it is that important.

The VCPR - Where You Stand and Where AI Does Not

The veterinarian-client-patient relationship, or VCPR, is the legal and ethical foundation of veterinary practice in the United States. The AVMA defines it as a relationship that exists when a veterinarian has assumed responsibility for making medical judgments about a patient, has sufficient knowledge of the patient to make a preliminary diagnosis, and is available for follow-up care.

The VCPR is yours. It cannot be transferred to a piece of software. It cannot be shared with a third-party AI platform. When you use AI to help draft a SOAP note or a client letter, you're using a writing tool. The clinical judgment in that document, the diagnosis, the treatment plan, the assessment of the patient's condition, that is yours, not the tool's.

The AVMA established a Task Force on Emerging Technologies and Innovation specifically to address the growing integration of AI into veterinary practice. As of this writing, the task force has been explicit: AI can support veterinary workflows, but it cannot hold the VCPR, and it cannot assume clinical responsibility. The veterinarian is and must remain the accountable party in every patient encounter.

This is not a technicality. At the 2025 AVMA Veterinary Business and Economic Forum, panelists from across the field discussed what they called "automation bias," the very human tendency to trust automated systems even when our own judgment would tell us otherwise. One panelist referenced aviation's experience with this problem directly: pilots who over-relied on autopilot systems lost the ability to catch errors those systems made. The same risk applies here. AI is a tool. It is not a colleague. It is not a consultant. It is not a second opinion. It is a very fast, very fluent text generator that needs your expert eye on everything it produces.

What Never Goes Into a Public AI Tool

This section is short because the rule is simple. When you are using a general consumer AI tool (ChatGPT, Claude, Gemini, or similar), you are sending text to a third-party server. What you type or paste becomes part of the conversation that the server processes. Depending on the tool's privacy settings, it may also be used to train future models.

That means the following never go into a public AI tool:

- Client full names
- Patient names combined with any identifying detail (species, owner name, address)
- Client contact information or addresses
- Account numbers or financial information
- Any detail that would allow a specific animal or owner to be identified from the text

Veterinary medicine is not subject to HIPAA. That law applies to human healthcare. But your state veterinary practice act almost certainly has confidentiality requirements that govern client and patient information. Your professional obligation to client privacy does not depend on a federal mandate.

The practical solution is de-identification, and it's faster than it sounds. Before you paste any clinical notes into an AI tool, you do a quick find-and-replace in your head: the patient becomes "a 7-year-old male neutered Labrador," not "Max Chen." The owner becomes "the client," not "Mrs. Chen." No address, no account number, no identifying detail. Just the clinical information.

We'll cover the de-identification workflow in detail in Chapter 3, and there is a printable quick-reference version in Appendix B. Once it becomes a habit, which takes about a week, it adds maybe ten seconds to each interaction.

The Hard Lines - What AI Never Does in Your Practice

Some applications of AI in veterinary medicine are not gray areas. They are clear limits, and you should have them written down somewhere before you start.

AI does not make clinical diagnoses. It can help you draft documentation of a diagnosis you've made. It can help you think through differentials as a sounding board, the way you might talk through a case with a colleague, but the clinical judgment is yours. Always.

AI does not touch your controlled substance logs. This one gets its own section later, but the short version is this: your DEA-required controlled substance records are legal documents with chain-of-custody requirements, signature verification, and reconciliation obligations. They must be accurate, they must be signed by authorized personnel, and a discrepancy in them can trigger a federal investigation. AI has no role in the actual log. Period. There are adjacent areas where AI can help, compliance policy documents, staff training materials, and audit preparation. We'll cover those. But the log itself is a human-only document.

AI does not replace your exam. This one should be obvious, but it needs saying. AI can help you document what you found. It cannot tell you what to find. The physical exam, the clinical reasoning, the assessment of the animal in front of you, that is medicine. That is why you have a license.

AI is not a drug reference. It can generate text that looks like a drug dosage calculation. It can be wrong. For any drug information that goes into a patient record or a client instruction, verify against a current, authoritative veterinary reference such as Plumb's, your formulary, or your PIMS drug database. Not the AI output.

Automation Bias - The Risk You Need to Know About

Here's a concern that doesn't get enough attention in most AI guides, and it is particularly important for veterinary medicine: the risk is not just that AI will make an error. The risk is that you'll stop catching the errors.

Humans are genuinely bad at sustained vigilance over automated systems. When something produces good output most of the time, we tend to trust it more over time. We skim instead of read. We approve instead of verify. This is documented extensively in aviation, in healthcare, and now in the early literature on AI-assisted clinical documentation.

At the 2025 AVMA Veterinary Business and Economic Forum, Dr. Petra Harms, founder and CEO of VetMaite, a veterinary AI consultancy and education platform, put it plainly: "It's not enough to have a human in the loop. It has to be an educated, confident human in the loop."

That means you need to be a careful, active reviewer of AI-generated content, not a rubber stamp. It means new graduates and early-career veterinarians, who may be building clinical habits while simultaneously using AI tools, need to be especially intentional about developing independent judgment.

And it means that the review step is not a formality. It is the job.

We'll come back to this in Chapter 4 when we get to SOAP notes specifically. For now, just know that this is on your radar.

Disclosure - Do You Tell Clients You Used AI?

This is a genuinely evolving question, and the honest answer is that clear professional consensus doesn't yet exist. The AVMA task force is working on guidance. State boards are beginning to address it. The landscape will be clearer in a few years than it is today.

Here's what we know as of this writing. Using AI to assist with documentation, the same way you might use a template, a voice recorder, or a scribe, is generally considered acceptable practice. Using AI in a way that materially affects clinical decision-making raises more significant questions about disclosure and consent.

The research supports a transparency-forward approach. A 2024 paper in JAVMA argued that when clinical decisions are influenced by AI systems, disclosure to clients engenders trust while keeping the veterinarian in an informed, accountable role. That is a reasonable standard to apply while formal guidance catches up.

A practical working policy: if a client asks whether you use AI tools, answer honestly. If AI assists in preparing a document the client receives, and they ask, say so. "I use AI to help draft some of our written communications and I review everything carefully before it goes out" is an accurate, professional, and trust-building answer.

You don't need to narrate your workflow on every discharge instruction. But if asked, be straight.

Building Your Personal AI Policy

This chapter ends with something practical rather than conceptual. Before you start using any of the techniques in this book, write down your own AI policy. It does not have to be long. It does not have to be formal. But having it written down, even in a note on your phone, does two things: it forces you to think through your own limits before you're in the middle of a busy clinic day, and it gives you something to refer to if a staff member or client ever asks.

Here's a simple framework:

What tools I will use: [List the specific tools you choose]

What I will use AI for:

- Drafting SOAP notes for my review
- Discharge instructions and client handouts
- Client communication letters
- Staff and operational documents
- Research and continuing education

What I will never use AI for:

- Clinical diagnosis or treatment decisions
- Controlled substance log entries
- Any document I will not personally review before it goes out

- Any input that contains client names, patient identifiers, or private information

My review process: Every AI-generated document that touches a patient or client will be read in full before I approve it, with specific attention to drug names, dosages, and any clinical recommendation.

That is it. One page. It shapes everything that follows.

A fillable version of this policy template is in Appendix D at the back of the book. Fill it in before you get to Chapter 3.

Chapter 2

The Paperwork Avalanche - Understanding Your Documentation Universe

Most veterinarians have never actually sat down and counted everything they write in a week. Not because they haven't noticed the volume, they definitely have, but because the documentation is so woven into the rhythm of the day that it becomes invisible. It's just the thing you do after every appointment, the thing you stay late to finish, the background hum of professional life.

Let's make it visible. Because before you can use AI to reduce your documentation burden, you need to understand the full scope of what you're actually producing. And the scope is larger than most people realize when they see it laid out.

This chapter maps your complete documentation universe, explains what is legally required in each area, and draws a clear line between where AI can help and where it cannot. That line is not an obstacle. It is the thing that makes the rest of the book trustworthy.

The Documents You Produce Every Single Day

SOAP Notes

The workhorse of veterinary documentation. SOAP stands for Subjective, Objective, Assessment, and Plan, and it's the gold standard format for clinical records in veterinary medicine. It is recommended by the AVMA, required by most state veterinary licensing boards to meet the standard of structured, problem-oriented medical records, and mandated for AAHA-accredited hospitals.

Here's what a complete SOAP note actually contains:

The Subjective section captures what the client reports: the chief complaint, the history of the current illness, behavior changes the owner has noticed, appetite and water intake, activity level, vaccination status, prior treatments tried at home, and relevant past medical history. It's the story of the visit from the client's perspective, filtered through your clinical eye.

The Objective section is everything measurable and observable from your exam: temperature, heart rate, respiratory rate, weight, body condition score, hydration status, mucous membrane color, capillary refill time, and a full system-by-system physical examination. Eyes, ears, oral cavity, lymph nodes, heart and lung sounds, abdominal palpation, musculoskeletal assessment, skin and coat condition, and neurologic status. Then diagnostic results: in-house bloodwork with reference ranges, pending lab submissions, radiograph or ultrasound findings, and urinalysis results. For controlled substances administered, the Objective section must include the exact dose in mg/kg, the total dose given, the route of administration, and the lot number from the clinic stock.

The Assessment section is your clinical reasoning made visible. It's where you synthesize the Subjective and Objective data into a working diagnosis or a ranked differential list, state your clinical rationale, note any diagnostic uncertainty, and document how the patient is responding to prior treatment if this is a recheck. This section is the legal record of your professional judgment.

The Plan section documents every next step: medications prescribed with exact dosages and duration, diagnostics ordered, surgical plans, referrals made, client education provided, and the follow-up schedule. The more specific this section is, the more useful it is for the next provider who sees the patient, and the more defensible it is if a question ever arises about the standard of care.

SOAP notes serve simultaneously as a clinical tool, a communication document for your team, a legal record in any malpractice proceeding, and supporting documentation for pet insurance claims. Sparse notes and brief entries without examination findings or diagnostic reasoning are a leading cause of pet insurance claim delays and denials, and they are among the most commonly cited deficiencies in state veterinary board disciplinary cases.

A routine wellness visit might be a single page. A complex multi-problem case might be two or three. The goal is not length, it is completeness of the clinical picture.

Where AI helps: drafting the narrative portions of the SOAP note from your bullet points or voice notes, especially the Subjective section and the Plan language. Where AI requires your careful verification: every drug name, dose, and route in the Objective and Plan sections. Where AI does not belong: the clinical Assessment. That is your diagnosis. You write that.

Discharge Instructions

Produced at virtually every appointment. For a wellness visit, this might be a vaccination summary and a brief wellness note. For a post-surgical patient, it's a detailed document covering wound care, activity restrictions, medication schedule with exact doses and timing, dietary changes, warning signs that require a call back, and follow-up appointment timing.

Discharge instructions are simultaneously a clinical document and a client communication tool, which means they need to be medically accurate and written in plain, warm language that a non-medical reader can follow while anxious about their pet. That combination is one of the harder writing challenges in practice and one that AI handles remarkably well when given good clinical input.

Where AI helps: almost everywhere. This is one of the highest-value use cases in the book.

Controlled Substance Logs

This section leads with the limit, because you need to know it immediately: AI does not touch your controlled substance log. Not to draft entries, not to help with reconciliation, not to fill in missing fields. The log is a legal document under the Controlled Substances Act and DEA regulations, and it has requirements that no AI tool can meet.

Here's what the law requires. Under 21 U.S.C. Section 821 and the associated DEA regulations, every veterinary practice registered to dispense or administer Schedule II through V controlled substances must maintain separate dispensing logs for each schedule. Every entry must record the date, patient name and species, drug name, strength, quantity administered or dispensed, the dose given, the route of administration, the balance remaining, and the name or initials of the authorized person who administered or dispensed. Entries must reconcile exactly with patient records. The DEA minimum retention requirement is two years. Many states require longer.

DEA audits cross-reference your drug log against your patient records and your on-hand inventory. A discrepancy, such as morphine logged as dispensed but with no corresponding patient record, or a running balance that does not match the physical count is not a paperwork error. It is a red flag that triggers formal investigation.

The log entries require verified signatures from authorized personnel. There's a chain of custody built into the system. No AI tool can sign a log, verify identity, or participate in that chain. It is a human-only process, and it needs to stay that way.

What AI can do in this area: help you draft your controlled substance compliance policy for staff, create training materials that walk new employees through logging procedures, prepare written summaries for your own internal audit prep, or draft the procedural SOPs that govern how your clinic handles controlled substances. The policy and the training around the log: that is AI territory. AI can even generate a blank log form with all of the required entries that you fill in. The log itself: never.

Surgical Reports and Anesthesia Records

Any invasive procedure generates documentation requirements beyond the standard SOAP note. A complete surgical record includes the pre-anesthetic evaluation (physical status, ASA classification, risk factors discussed with client), the anesthetic protocol (pre-medications, induction agents, maintenance, monitoring equipment used), intraoperative notes (duration, complications, monitoring values at intervals), and recovery documentation (time to sternal, extubation, discharge criteria met). Controlled substances used during anesthesia must be documented in both the anesthesia record and the controlled substance log, with reconciliation between the two.

These records are legal documents. In a malpractice claim, the anesthesia record is often the first thing examined.

Where AI helps: drafting the narrative portions of post-surgical client communication, writing post-operative care instructions, and helping create standardized templates for your anesthesia record structure.

Referral Letters and Specialist Correspondence

When you transfer care to a specialist or an emergency facility, the AVMA guidelines specify that records should accompany the referral or be transmitted promptly on request. A referral letter needs to summarize the patient's history, your findings, the diagnostics you've run, your working diagnosis, what you've already tried, and the specific reason for referral. It needs to be clear, thorough, and professional, because the specialist is making decisions based on what you give them.

These letters are time-consuming to write well, and they often get written at the end of a difficult day after a hard case. AI is good at this. Give it your clinical bullet points and it will give you a polished, professional referral letter to review and send.

Treatment Sheets for Hospitalized Patients

When a patient stays in the hospital, documentation shifts from a single encounter note to a continuous, shift-spanning record. Treatment sheets log vital signs at regular intervals, medication administrations with exact timing and initials, fluid rates, nursing observations, and changes in patient status throughout the hospitalization. They're updated by multiple staff members across multiple shifts.

The treatment sheet is the source document for the discharge SOAP note. The final note draws on the accumulated data in the treatment sheet to summarize the patient's course of care and document the discharge plan.

Where AI helps: drafting the discharge summary narrative, creating standardized treatment sheet templates, and generating the discharge instructions that go home with the client at the end of the hospitalization.

Vaccine and Wellness Records

Vaccination records are required by law for rabies in every state and are essential documentation for boarding facilities, groomers, travel certificates, and legal proceedings. A complete vaccine record includes the vaccine name, manufacturer, lot number, expiration date, date administered, route and site, and the administering provider. These are typically managed within your PIMS, but the underlying documentation requirements are legal ones.

Estimate and Financial Documentation

Treatment estimates, signed consent forms, and the documented record of financial discussions with clients are part of the medical record in a meaningful legal sense. Incomplete financial documentation such as an estimate that was never signed, a consent form that is missing, or a financial conversation that was never noted creates real liability exposure in disputed cases. Pet insurance providers also require clear documentation of the treatment plan and associated costs to process reimbursement.

Where AI helps: drafting estimate language, writing treatment plan summaries, and creating templated consent form language for common procedures.

Client Communication Records

Phone calls, follow-up emails, and client education provided during a visit are part of the clinical picture and should be noted in the record. "Client called, advised to bring patient in if vomiting continues" is a one-line note, but in a malpractice proceeding it can be the difference between a defensible record and an indefensible one.

Where AI helps: drafting follow-up email templates for common scenarios, writing standard callback language for common post-procedure concerns.

The Numbers Behind the Burden

Now you can see why the numbers are what they are. A 2025 FVE report found that 64% of veterinarians reported their administrative workload had doubled. This makes more sense when you can see everything that falls under "administrative work." It is not one thing. It is a dozen distinct document types, each with its own requirements, its own legal weight, and its own time cost.

The same FVE report found that practices report DVMs and support staff spending multiple unpaid hours daily on charts alone. The single most time-consuming documentation category was prescribing and dispensing. This consumed up to ten hours per week for many veterinarians. Ten hours that mostly happen after the last patient leaves and mostly go uncompensated.

That is the problem this book is here to address. The goal is not to eliminate documentation. The goal should be making the writable parts of it faster and better so the hours you spend on patient care and your own life are protected.

Your Documentation Map

Here's a simple reference to carry forward as you read the rest of this book. For each document type, the table below shows what AI can help with and where the hard limits are.

Document Type	AI Can Help	AI Hard Limit
SOAP notes	Drafting Subjective and Plan narrative	Clinical Assessment: that is your diagnosis
Discharge instructions	Full draft from clinical bullets	Verify all drug names, doses, and timing
Controlled substance logs	Policy docs, training materials, audit prep	The actual log entries: human only
Surgical/anesthesia records	Post-op client communication, templates	The clinical record requires your review
Referral letters	Full draft from clinical bullets	Verify all clinical details before sending
Treatment sheets	Discharge summary, client instructions	All medication entries need human verification
Client communication	Full drafts, templates	Always review before sending
Financial/consent docs	Estimate language, consent templates	Signed consent requires human process

Print that. Tape it up somewhere. It is the frame for everything that follows.

Chapter 3

Getting Started Without Feeling Overwhelmed

You don't need a technology background to use AI tools effectively. You don't need to understand how they work under the hood any more than you need to understand combustion engines to drive a car. What you need is a practical orientation, an understanding of what the main tools are, how to access them, how to talk to them in a way that gets useful results, and what a first session actually looks like.

That is the goal of this chapter. We're going to keep it direct and get you to your first useful output as quickly as possible.

The Four Tools Worth Knowing

There are many AI tools on the market. For the purposes of this book, four are worth your attention as starting points: ChatGPT (made by OpenAI), Claude (made by Anthropic), Gemini (made by Google) and Grok (made by xAI). All four are accessible through a web browser or a phone app. All four have free tiers that will let you start without spending anything.

ChatGPT is the most widely known and has been around the longest. It is strong on general writing tasks, familiar to most people who have experimented with AI at all, and integrates with several veterinary PIMS and documentation tools that are building AI features into their platforms. The free tier is capable. The paid tier (currently around $20 a month) gives you access to a more powerful version of the model and more reliable performance during peak hours.

Claude tends to produce particularly natural-sounding prose and handles nuanced instructions well. If you give it detailed guidance about tone and context, it tends to follow that guidance more precisely than some other tools. It is also conservative about generating medical content it is uncertain about, which in a clinical writing context can actually be a feature rather than a bug. Free tier available; paid tier similar pricing to ChatGPT.

Gemini is Google's offering and integrates with Google Workspace. If your practice uses Gmail and Google Docs, there is a reasonable case for Gemini because of that integration. Quality has improved significantly in recent iterations.

Grok is developed by xAI and is available through the X platform. It tends toward a more direct, conversational tone than the other major tools and has real-time access to information posted on X, which occasionally makes it useful for quickly surfacing current discussions in a field. For veterinary documentation workflows it performs competently on standard writing tasks. Free tier available through X; paid tier bundled with X Premium.

For starting out, use whichever one you're drawn to. The techniques in this book work with all four. The prompts in Chapter 11 are written to be tool-agnostic. Pick one, open an account, and use it for a few weeks before deciding whether you want to try another. The learning curve is the same across tools, and consistency matters more than which tool you chose.

A note on purpose-built veterinary AI tools. There is a growing category of AI tools designed specifically for veterinary documentation. They consist of products like CoVet, HappyDoc, and Acorn.vet, among others. These tools integrate directly with your PIMS, use ambient listening to capture exam room conversations, and generate SOAP notes automatically from what they hear. They are worth knowing about and some practices are getting excellent results with them. They are also a separate category from what this book primarily covers, which are general-purpose AI tools you can start using today for free. Appendix C has a current overview of the veterinary-specific tool landscape if you want to explore that direction.

Free Versus Paid - What You Actually Get

The free tiers of all four major tools are genuinely capable. For the workflows in this book (drafting SOAP notes, writing discharge instructions, generating client letters) you can accomplish a great deal without spending anything. The main limitations of free tiers are response speed during busy periods, occasional limits on how much you can generate per day, and access to the most advanced version of the model.

The paid tiers (typically around $20 per month) give you faster responses, higher daily limits, and access to more capable model versions that handle complex instructions better. For a practicing veterinarian using AI as a regular part of their workflow, $20 a month is a reasonable expense that will pay for itself quickly in time saved.

Start free. If you find yourself bumping into limits or wanting better performance after a few weeks, upgrade. There's no reason to spend money before you know how much you'll use it.

The Cardinal Privacy Rule in Practice

Chapter 1 established the rule: no client names, no patient identifiers, no private information in a public AI tool. Here's what that looks like in the actual workflow.

You finish an exam. Your notes look something like this in your head, or in a quick phone voice memo:

"Max Chen, 7-year-old MN Lab, presented for vomiting x 3 days. Owner says he got into the trash four days ago. Eating some, drinking well. No blood in vomit. On exam: mild cranial abdominal pain on palpation, otherwise unremarkable. BCS 5/9, temp 102.1, HR 88, RR 24. CBC/chem panel pending. Started on Cerenia 60mg SQ, sent home with metronidazole 500mg BID x 5 days and bland diet. Recheck if not improving in 48 hours or if vomiting worsens."

Before that goes into an AI tool, you do a ten-second mental find-and-replace:

"Max Chen" becomes "a 7-year-old male neutered Labrador."

"Owner" stays "the owner." No name.

Everything else in those notes is clinical information, not identifying information.

Your de-identified version: "7-year-old male neutered Labrador presented for vomiting x 3 days following possible dietary indiscretion. Owner reports some food intake, normal water consumption, no hematochezia or hematemesis. Physical exam findings: mild cranial abdominal pain on deep palpation, otherwise within normal limits. TPR within normal range.

CBC/chemistry panel pending. Administered Cerenia 60mg SQ. Dispensed metronidazole 500mg BID x 5 days and recommended bland diet. Client advised to return if not improving in 48 hours or if vomiting worsens."

That took about fifteen seconds. That de-identified version is what goes into the AI tool. Everything about the clinical picture is there. Nothing about the client or patient is identifiable.

The detailed de-identification workflow and a printable quick-reference card are in Appendix B.

Prompting Basics - Asking Good Questions Gets Good Answers

A prompt is just what you type into the AI tool. Better prompts get better results. It's not complicated, but there are a few principles worth knowing before you start.

Be specific about what you want. "Write a SOAP note" will get you a generic result. "Write the Subjective and Plan sections of a veterinary SOAP note for a 7-year-old male neutered Labrador presenting for vomiting following possible dietary indiscretion. The owner reports some food intake, normal water consumption, and no blood in the vomit. The plan includes Cerenia 60mg SQ in clinic, metronidazole 500mg BID x 5 days dispensed, bland diet recommended, and recheck in 48 hours if not improving" will get you something you can actually use.

Tell the tool who it is writing for. "Write discharge instructions for the owner of a post-surgical dog" is okay. "Write discharge instructions for a pet owner in warm, clear, non-medical language, for a dog that had an uncomplicated splenectomy this morning" is a significantly better prompt and will give a significantly better output.

Give it the clinical details upfront. AI tools do not go looking for information. They work with what you give them. The more complete your clinical input, the more complete and accurate the output.

Tell it the format you want. "Write this as a bulleted list" or "write this as two short paragraphs" or "write this in the format of a professional referral letter" all of this detail will help the tool give you an output that fits your workflow.

Iterate. Your first result will often be close but not quite right. It's easier to refine a draft than to start from scratch. "Make this warmer in tone" or "shorten this to one paragraph" or "add a section about when to call the clinic" are all simple follow-up prompts that get you to a better result without starting over.

Your First Session - A Real Walkthrough

Here's a complete first session so you can see how this actually flows. Use this as a practice run before you bring it into your real clinic workflow.

Open whichever tool you've chosen. You're going to paste in a de-identified clinical scenario and ask for a SOAP note draft.

Type or paste the following prompt:

"You are helping a veterinarian draft clinical documentation. Write the Subjective and Plan sections of a veterinary SOAP note for the following case. Use professional veterinary language. Be thorough in the Plan section, including medication names, doses, routes, and client instructions.

Patient: 4-year-old female spayed domestic shorthair cat

Chief complaint: Straining to urinate, crying in the litter box, x 24 hours

History: Indoor only, no prior urinary issues. Eating and drinking normally until yesterday. No vomiting. Current on vaccines and monthly flea prevention.

Physical exam findings: Mild discomfort on caudal abdominal palpation, bladder small and expressible, no urethral obstruction. Otherwise within normal limits. Temperature 102.3, HR 172, RR 28, weight 4.1 kg.

Diagnostics: Urinalysis pending.

Plan: Buprenorphine 0.01 mg/kg SQ administered in clinic for pain management. Dispensed meloxicam 0.05 mg/kg PO SID x 3 days. Recommended increased water intake, wet food diet. Urinalysis pending. Client to call for results. Recheck in 5 days or sooner if straining worsens or patient stops urinating."

Hit send. Read what you get. Then try a follow-up: "Rewrite the Plan section so it reads as instructions the owner will take home -- clear, simple language, no abbreviations."

Notice how the second version is different. Notice what the tool got right and what you would change if this were a real patient. That review instinct, the active reading of the output, is the skill you're building.

Do this a few more times with different scenarios before you bring AI into your real workflow. The tool will feel less foreign after two or three practice runs, and you'll have a much better sense of how to prompt it effectively for your specific documentation style.

In Chapter 4, we go deeper into SOAP notes specifically, with species-specific prompts, multi-problem case handling, and a full prompt library for your most common presentations. By the end of that chapter, you'll have everything you need to start using AI in real cases.

For now: open the tool, try the walkthrough above, and get a feel for what you're working with.

The rest gets easier from here.

Chapter 4

SOAP Notes - Getting Two Hours Back Every Day

Let's talk about where your time actually goes.

If you're a full-time small animal practitioner seeing 20 to 30 patients a day, you're writing 20 to 30 SOAP notes. Some of those are straightforward: a wellness visit, a vaccine recheck, a suture removal. Some are not. A complex multi-problem geriatric patient, a diagnostic workup that ran three directions at once, an emergency that came in sideways and kept you on your feet for an hour. By the time you get to the notes on those cases, it's often late, you're tired, and the clinical details you want to capture are already starting to blur together.

This is where documentation quality quietly erodes. Not through carelessness, but through fatigue and time pressure. The note that should be thorough becomes a shorthand sketch. The clinical reasoning that should be visible in the Assessment gets compressed into a single line. The Plan section that should give your associate everything they need at a recheck becomes a list of medications without context.

AI does not replace your clinical judgment. It does not think about your patient. But it's genuinely excellent at one specific job: taking your clinical bullet points and turning them into well-structured, professionally written documentation that you can review, correct, and finalize in a fraction of the time it would take to write from scratch.

Veterinarians using AI documentation tools report cutting their documentation time by 40% to 75%. Even at the conservative end of that range, on a day with 25 patients, that's real time returned to you, time for patients, for clients, for the walk to your car before it gets dark.

Here is how to do it.

The Core Workflow - Bullet Points In, Draft Out

The workflow is simpler than most people expect. It has four steps.

Step 1: Capture your clinical notes during or immediately after the exam. This can be a voice memo on your phone, a few quick bullet points in your PIMS, or a handwritten note on a scratch pad. The goal is to capture the clinical details while they're fresh and to get the raw information down, not to write the full SOAP note. Speed matters here more than completeness. You can fill gaps from memory when you review, but you cannot recover details you never captured.

Step 2: De-identify your notes. Take 10 seconds to swap out identifying details before anything goes into an AI tool. The patient's name becomes a signalment. The owner's name becomes "the client." The de-identification workflow is in Appendix B if you need a quick reference until it becomes a habit.

Step 3: Paste your de-identified notes into the AI tool with a clear prompt. Tell the tool what you want, what the patient is, and what format you need. The prompts at the end of this chapter and in Chapter 11 are ready to copy and use.

Step 4: Review and finalize. Read the output. Fix anything that's wrong. Pay specific attention to drug names, doses, routes, and any clinical recommendation. The review is not optional and is not a formality. It is the job. What you approve goes into the record. Your name is on it.

That is the whole workflow. The rest of this chapter is about making each step faster and more reliable for the specific cases you see every day.

Writing Prompts That Get Good Results

The quality of what comes out is directly related to the quality of what goes in. Here's the prompt structure that works consistently for SOAP note drafting:

"You are helping a veterinarian draft a clinical SOAP note. Using the information below, write the [Subjective / Plan / full SOAP note] section in professional veterinary language. Be specific about medications including names, doses, routes, and frequency. Do not invent clinical details that are not provided.

[Paste your de-identified clinical notes here]"

That structure does three things: it establishes context (veterinary clinical writing), it specifies what you want (which section or all sections), and it gives the tool an important instruction at the end (do not invent details). That last line matters. Without it, some AI tools will occasionally fill gaps by guessing, and a plausible-sounding but invented detail in a clinical record is a problem.

A few refinements that make a real difference:

"Write the Assessment section as a differential diagnosis list with the most likely diagnosis first, followed by the clinical rationale" tells the tool exactly what format you want for that section.

"Write the Plan section so it can be read by a veterinary technician -- clear, specific, and in the order the tasks should be completed" shifts the writing toward a more usable clinical handoff document.

"This is a recheck appointment. The patient was last seen 10 days ago for [condition]. The Plan from the previous visit was [brief summary]. Write the Subjective section reflecting the client's update on how the patient has responded" gives the tool the context it needs to write a coherent progress note rather than a first-visit note.

Species-Specific Considerations

The AI tools available today were trained on a much larger pool of canine and feline content than any other species. That means they write confidently about dogs and cats, and you should be more careful with their output on anything else. Chapter 8 covers exotics and large animals in detail. For now, a few notes for the cases that come up most in mixed practice:

For feline patients, always verify dosing and drug selection independently. Cats have well-documented drug metabolism differences: acetaminophen toxicity, NSAIDs, certain antibiotics and, and opioid sensitivities. AI tools handle these inconsistently. Never let an AI-generated Plan section for a cat go out without checking every drug against a current feline formulary.

For equine patients, normal vital sign ranges, drug dosages, and clinical findings are different enough from companion animals that AI output on equine cases should be treated with extra scrutiny. Provide the normal ranges you expect when writing equine prompts, or verify all values independently.

For pocket pets, birds, and reptiles, assume the tool's training data is thin and verify everything clinical. Use AI for the writing and structure of these notes, but apply your own knowledge and training to every clinical detail.

Multi-Problem Cases

Some of your most time-consuming documentation is the complex multi-problem patient: the 12-year-old dog with osteoarthritis, hypothyroidism, a new skin mass that needs monitoring, and mild dental disease found incidentally during the exam. The SOAP note for that patient needs to address each problem with its own Assessment and Plan, and keeping the documentation organized and clear is a genuine challenge.

AI handles multi-problem cases well if you give it a clear structure. Here's how to frame the prompt:

"Write a SOAP note for a multi-problem patient. Address each problem in the Assessment and Plan sections separately, clearly labeled. The problems are:

Problem 1: [Describe]

Problem 2: [Describe]

Problem 3: [Describe]

Patient information: [De-identified signalment and clinical findings]"

The output will typically be organized by problem in the Assessment and Plan sections, which both matches the Problem-Oriented Medical Record format and makes the note far more useful for whoever sees the patient next.

The Review Step - What to Check Every Time

The review is where your clinical expertise protects your patients and your license. Here's a specific checklist for reviewing AI-generated SOAP notes:

Drug names: correct spelling, correct drug, nothing invented or substituted. AI tools occasionally suggest a drug that is close to what you specified but is not quite right.

Dosages: verify every dose against your own knowledge or a current reference. Confirm the dose is appropriate for this patient's weight and species. Confirm the route is correct.

Clinical details: make sure the AI has not invented findings. If your Objective section says the abdominal palpation was unremarkable, confirm the AI did not add a detail that was not in your notes.

Assessment accuracy: your diagnosis is your diagnosis. Make sure the Assessment reflects what you actually think, not a reasonable guess the AI made based on the Subjective and Objective.

Plan completeness: confirm everything that happened and everything you recommended is in the Plan. Confirm nothing is missing.

Tone and language: confirm the note sounds like your practice's documentation style. You have the right to fix wording, shorten things, or expand where needed.

This review takes two to three minutes on a typical case. On a complex case, it might take five. That is still far less than writing from scratch, and the review builds the habit of active, critical engagement with AI output that protects you from automation bias over time.

Case Study: A Complete SOAP Note, From Exam to Record

The best way to see how this workflow actually runs is to watch one go from start to finish. Here's a real-world style case, start to end.

Midday appointment, walk-in, visibly distressed owner. A cat has been vomiting for two days and is now lethargic. The exam takes twenty minutes. You finish, give your working diagnosis, start treatment, and walk the client out. Your next appointment is in five minutes.

Here's what you would have captured if you were writing this SOAP note longhand, the old way.

Your raw clinical notes (captured as a voice memo, then transcribed):

9yo FS DSH, vomiting x2 days, now lethargic, not eating since yesterday evening. Owner reports 3 episodes today, yellow bile. No blood. Indoor only, no known toxin exposure, no access to string or plants. Last normal meal Tuesday night. On exam: BCS 5/9, mildly dehydrated approx 5%, tacky MM, mild abdominal discomfort on deep palpation, no palpable foreign body, no organomegaly. Temp 102.8, HR 200, RR 32. Recommended bloodwork and radiographs. CBC showed mild left shift, chem panel within normal limits. Radiographs unremarkable, no foreign body visible. Started on IV fluids 60ml/hr, Cerenia 1mg/kg SQ, famotidine 0.5mg/kg IV. Plan to hospitalize overnight for continued fluids and monitoring. Will recheck in the morning. If not improving by tomorrow AM, will pursue abdominal ultrasound.

That is your actual thinking, captured fast, slightly fragmented, and not in any shape to go into a record.

Step 1: de-identify.

Take ten seconds. The patient has no identifying name in the raw notes, which is already good habit. No owner name appears. Nothing to remove. These notes are ready.

Step 2: the prompt.

Paste the following into your AI tool:

"You are helping a veterinarian draft a clinical SOAP note. Write the complete SOAP note using the information below. Use professional veterinary language. Be specific about all medications including doses in mg/kg where relevant, total doses, routes, and frequency. Do not add clinical details that are not provided. Flag any section where you are uncertain rather than guessing."

Followed by the raw clinical notes from above.

Step 3: the AI's draft.

Here's what came back.

S (Subjective): Nine-year-old female spayed domestic shorthair presenting for vomiting of two days' duration with progressive lethargy. Owner reports three episodes of yellow bilious emesis today, no hematemesis noted. Patient has been anorexic since Tuesday evening. Indoor-only cat with no known toxin exposure and no reported access to foreign material including string or plants.

O (Objective): Alert but subdued on presentation. BCS 5/9. Mild dehydration estimated at approximately 5% based on tacky mucous membranes. Temperature 102.8, heart rate 200 bpm, respiratory rate 32. Abdominal palpation revealed mild discomfort on deep palpation with no palpable foreign body or organomegaly. CBC: mild left shift. Chemistry panel: within normal limits. Abdominal radiographs: unremarkable, no foreign body identified.

A (Assessment): Feline gastroenteritis, etiology undetermined. Differential considerations include dietary indiscretion, infectious gastroenteritis, and early-stage obstructive process despite unremarkable imaging. Mild dehydration secondary to fluid losses and decreased intake.

P (Plan): Hospitalized for IV fluid therapy at 60 mL/hr. Administered maropitant citrate (Cerenia) 1 mg/kg SQ for antiemetic support. Famotidine 0.5 mg/kg IV for gastric acid suppression. NPO overnight with plan to reassess in the morning. If clinical signs do not improve by AM, abdominal ultrasound will be pursued to rule out occult obstructive or infiltrative process.

Step 4: your review.

Read the whole draft with your clinical eye. Here's what you catch.

Drug names and doses: all three correct. Cerenia (maropitant) 1 mg/kg SQ, famotidine 0.5 mg/kg IV. Verify against your formulary anyway.

The Assessment section is yours to confirm. The AI gave a reasonable differential, but the word "undetermined" is doing work. You believe this is most likely dietary-indiscretion gastroenteritis; change "etiology undetermined" to "most consistent with dietary indiscretion gastroenteritis, with obstructive process not yet fully excluded."

The Plan is accurate but misses one detail from your notes: you wanted to recheck in the morning specifically before any additional diagnostics, and the plan should reflect that sequencing. Add a sentence: "Morning recheck will include repeat physical exam, assessment of hydration, and check for any clinical improvement before pursuing further diagnostics."

One thing to add that you mentioned in the exam but not in your voice memo: the client declined pet insurance coverage for the hospitalization and was counseled on signs that would prompt an earlier call. That conversation happened and should be in the record. Add a one-line client communication note to the Plan.

Step 5: the finalized note.

Your edited version goes into the patient record. Total time from exam end to finalized SOAP note: about five minutes. Three of those were you reading and editing. Two were the AI drafting while you grabbed a quick sip of water between appointments.

The old way, writing this from scratch at 7:30 that night after your last patient left? Fifteen to twenty minutes.

This is not a system where the AI writes your record and you sign it. It is a system where the AI drafts, you edit, and your clinical judgment is visible in every edit. That is the same relationship you have with a scribe, except faster, and you can do it yourself at 2pm between appointments instead of at 9pm at home.

Prompt Library - SOAP Notes

The following prompts are ready to copy and use. Each can be pasted directly into any major AI tool with your de-identified clinical details filled in.

General SOAP Note - Full Draft

"You are helping a veterinarian document a patient visit. Write a complete SOAP note using the clinical information below. Use professional veterinary language. Be specific about all medications including generic names, doses in mg/kg where relevant, total doses, routes, and frequency. Do not add clinical details that are not provided. Flag any section where you are uncertain rather than guessing.

[Paste de-identified clinical notes]"

Subjective Section Only

"Write the Subjective section of a veterinary SOAP note based on the following owner-reported history and chief complaint. Capture the key clinical history in professional language. Patient is [signalment].

[Paste de-identified owner history and chief complaint]"

Plan Section - Clinician Use

"Write the Plan section of a veterinary SOAP note for the following case. Include all medications with doses, routes, and frequency. Include diagnostics ordered, follow-up timing, and client instructions provided. Use professional veterinary clinical language. Do not add clinical details that are not provided.

[Paste de-identified plan details]"

Plan Section - Technician Handoff Format

"Write the Plan section of a veterinary SOAP note formatted as a clear technician task list. Organize by task order. Include all medications with doses, routes, and frequency. Be specific enough that a veterinary technician can execute the plan without asking for clarification.

[Paste de-identified plan details]"

Recheck / Progress Note

"This is a recheck visit. Write the Subjective section as a progress note. The patient was previously treated for [condition] with the following plan: [brief prior plan summary]. Today the owner reports the following: [de-identified owner update]. Patient is [signalment]."

Multi-Problem Case

"Write the Assessment and Plan sections of a SOAP note for a patient with multiple active problems. Address each problem separately with its own Assessment and Plan, clearly labeled. Patient is [signalment].

Problem 1: [Description and relevant findings]

Problem 2: [Description and relevant findings]

Problem 3: [Description and relevant findings]"

Chapter 5

Discharge Instructions and Client Handouts

Here's a piece of information that veterinary practice management consultants cite regularly and that most clinicians feel instinctively: client compliance with home care instructions is one of the most significant factors in patient outcomes. And client compliance is directly tied to how clearly those instructions are written.

A discharge document that is technically correct but written in clinical shorthand is not actually useful to the person reading it at home at 10pm, wondering whether the amount of drainage from the incision they're looking at is normal or not. A document that is warm, clear, specific, and written to anticipate the questions the client will actually have. That one gets followed.

Writing that kind of document from scratch, for every patient, every day, is genuinely time-consuming. It requires you to translate clinical thinking into plain language, to anticipate the worried owner rather than the informed colleague, and to do it with a level of care that's hard to sustain across 25 patients on a busy Wednesday.

This is the application where AI delivers the most consistent, immediately usable results. Give it your clinical details and the right instruction, and it will give you a polished, warm, readable discharge document in under two minutes. You review it, adjust anything specific to this patient, and it goes out. That is the workflow.

What Good Discharge Instructions Actually Contain

Before we get to the prompts, let's be clear about what thorough discharge instructions include, because what you give the AI to work with determines what you get back.

A complete discharge document contains the following:

The diagnosis or working diagnosis in plain language, not the ICD code, not the clinical shorthand, but the actual explanation of what's going on with this animal.

The treatment administered in the clinic: what was done, in language the owner can understand and repeat back to another vet if needed.

The medications going home: for each medication, the name (both brand and generic if possible), the dose in practical terms (how many pills, how much liquid), the frequency, the duration, what it's for, and how to give it. Not just "Metronidazole 250mg BID x 7 days." A client needs to know what that means in their kitchen at 7am.

Activity restrictions: specific and time-bound. "Rest" means nothing. "No running, jumping, or climbing stairs for 10 days" means something.

Dietary instructions: if applicable, what to feed, how much, for how long, and what to avoid.

Wound care instructions: if applicable, what normal healing looks like, how to clean, when to check, what to leave alone.

Warning signs that require a call or a return visit: specific, not vague. Not "if you notice any changes." List the actual signs: vomiting more than twice in 24 hours, temperature over 104, wound that opens or smells different, not eating for more than 48 hours.

Follow-up plan: when to return, what will be assessed, what happens next.

Contact information: clinic phone number and what to do outside of business hours.

That is the full document. When you prompt an AI tool, give it all of that information in your clinical notes and it will organize it into a readable, well-structured handout.

The Core Discharge Prompt

"Write discharge instructions for a pet owner. Use warm, clear, non-medical language that is easy to understand and follow at home. Avoid clinical abbreviations. Organize with clear section headers. The patient is [signalment -- species, breed, age, sex].

Diagnosis / reason for visit: [Plain language description]

Treatment provided today: [What was done]

Medications going home:

- [Drug name, dose in practical terms, frequency, duration, purpose]

- [Repeat for each medication]

Activity restrictions: [Specific restrictions and duration]

Diet: [If applicable]

Wound/incision care: [If applicable]

Warning signs to watch for and when to call: [List specific signs]

Follow-up: [When and why]

Clinic contact: [Your clinic name and phone -- add after AI generates the document]"

That structure gives the tool everything it needs. The output will typically be a well-organized, client-ready document that needs a quick read and minor personalization before it goes out.

Post-Surgical Discharge Instructions

Surgical patients need the most detailed and specific discharge documents, and they're the ones most likely to generate after-hours calls when the instructions are unclear. A thorough post-surgical discharge document practically eliminates the "is this normal?" calls and replaces them with owner confidence.

For a surgical patient, your prompt should specifically include:

The procedure performed and what was found, in plain language.

Incision location and what it looks like now, so the owner knows what they're monitoring.

What normal healing looks like at 24 hours, at 48 hours, at day 5, at day 10. Specific milestones help owners feel informed rather than anxious.

E-collar instructions: when to use it, what happens if they don't, how long.

Specific warning signs for surgical patients: incision opening, discharge that's yellow or foul-smelling, excessive swelling, patient not eating 24 hours post-surgery, breathing changes (for thoracic or certain abdominal procedures).

"Write detailed post-surgical discharge instructions for a pet owner. Warm, clear, plain language. The patient is [signalment].

Procedure performed: [Description in plain language]

What was found: [If applicable - e.g., mass removed, intestinal foreign body retrieved]

Incision location and current appearance: [Describe]

Pain medication going home: [Name, dose in practical terms, frequency, duration]

Other medications: [List if applicable]

E-collar: [Yes/no, how long, why]

Activity restrictions: [Specific and time-bound]

Diet tonight and tomorrow: [What and how much]

What normal healing looks like over the next 10 days: [Key milestones]

Warning signs that require a call: [List specific signs]

Suture removal / recheck appointment: [When and what will happen]"

Chronic Disease Management Handouts

Clients managing a pet with a chronic condition (diabetes, hypothyroidism, chronic kidney disease, Cushing's disease, Addison's disease, heart disease) benefit enormously from a clear, comprehensive handout they can refer to at home. These documents go beyond a single-visit discharge instruction. They become a reference the owner returns to.

Building a library of these handouts for your practice's most common chronic conditions is one of the highest-value things you can do with a single AI session. Write them once, review them carefully, and use them for every appropriate patient from that point forward.

The prompt for a chronic disease handout:

"Write a comprehensive home care guide for a pet owner whose dog/cat has been diagnosed with [condition]. The owner is motivated but has no medical background. The guide should cover:

What [condition] is and what causes it: brief, plain language

How it affects the pet day-to-day: what the owner will notice

The treatment plan: [List medications, doses in practical terms, monitoring schedule]

How to monitor at home: specific signs of good control vs. signs of a problem

What to do if they miss a dose

Dietary requirements: [Specify]

Exercise guidelines: [Specify]

Follow-up schedule: [What tests, how often, what you are checking]

Questions to bring to the next appointment

Keep the tone warm and empowering, because this owner is going to be their pet's primary caregiver. They need confidence, not anxiety."

This prompt reliably produces a document that's worth keeping and refining. Review it carefully, especially any clinical guidance on monitoring values and signs of crisis, which you should verify against your own clinical standards.

Specific Prompts for Common Presentations

The following are ready-to-use prompts for discharge situations that come up in virtually every small animal practice. Fill in the bracketed fields with your patient's specifics.

Post-Spay / Neuter

"Write discharge instructions for a pet owner after their [dog/cat] was spayed/neutered today. Patient is [signalment]. Anesthesia was uneventful. E-collar provided. Home with [pain medication name, dose, frequency, duration]. Activity restriction: [duration]. Suture removal in [X] days. Warning signs: incision opening, swelling, excessive licking, lethargy beyond 24 hours, not eating beyond 24 hours, discharge from incision site."

Acute Gastroenteritis / Dietary Indiscretion

"Write discharge instructions for the owner of a [dog/cat] seen for vomiting and/or diarrhea. Patient is [signalment]. [Diagnosis/working diagnosis in plain language]. Medications going home: [list with practical doses/frequency]. Dietary instructions: [bland diet, how long, how to transition back]. Warning signs to call: vomiting more than twice in 24 hours, blood in stool or vomit, lethargy, not improving after 48 hours. Recheck if not improving."

Skin / Ear Condition

"Write discharge instructions for the owner of a [dog/cat] treated for [skin/ear condition]. Patient is [signalment]. Treatment today: [what was done]. Medications going home: [list with practical doses, frequency, application instructions if topical]. What the owner will see as it improves. How long before they should see improvement. Warning signs. Follow-up at [timeframe]."

Post-Dental Procedure

"Write discharge instructions for the owner of a [dog/cat] who had a dental cleaning [with/without extractions] today. Patient is [signalment]. Extractions: [list sites if applicable]. Soft food for [X] days. Pain medication: [name, dose, frequency, duration]. No chew toys or hard treats for [X] days. What to expect -- mild facial swelling is normal, blood-tinged saliva for 24 hours is normal. Warning signs: not eating after 48 hours, persistent bleeding, pawing at mouth. Recheck at [timeframe]."

Urinary Tract Infection

"Write discharge instructions for the owner of a [dog/cat] diagnosed with a urinary tract infection. Patient is [signalment]. Antibiotic going home: [name, dose in practical terms, frequency, duration]. Importance of completing the full course. Signs of improvement to watch for. Signs that it is not improving -- still straining, blood in urine after 5 days, lethargy, not eating. Recheck urinalysis at [timeframe]."

Case Study: A Post-Surgical Discharge Document That Gets Followed

The gap between a technically accurate discharge instruction and one that actually gets followed is larger than most clinicians realize. Here's a complete case showing that gap closed.

The patient: a six-year-old male neutered Golden Retriever. Today's procedure: laparoscopic gastropexy as a prophylactic measure given breed risk for GDV. Uncomplicated surgery, routine recovery. Owner is a first-time large-breed owner, attentive but anxious, asked three questions during the pre-surgical consult.

Your clinical notes for the discharge document:

Procedure: elective laparoscopic gastropexy. Three small incisions right lateral abdomen, 5mm each, closed with intradermal sutures and skin glue. No intraoperative complications. Recovery uneventful. E-collar dispensed. Home on gabapentin 10mg/kg PO q8h x 5 days for pain management, carprofen 2mg/kg PO q12h x 7 days. Activity restriction: leash walks only, no running/jumping/stair climbing for 10 days. Soft food tonight, normal diet tomorrow. Warning signs for owner: incision opening or discharge, refusing food beyond 24 hours, vomiting, excessive swelling at incision site, lethargy beyond 24 hours post-surgery. Recheck in 10 days for incision assessment.

Step 1: de-identify.

Patient signalment is fine to include (species, breed, age, sex). No owner name in the notes. Ready.

Step 2: the prompt.

You use the Post-Surgical Discharge prompt from Chapter 11, filling in the clinical details from your notes and adding one context line at the top: "This is the owner's first large-breed dog and they're attentive but anxious." That one sentence shapes the tone of the entire document.

Step 3: the AI's draft.

What comes back is a seven-section document organized with clear headers. A sample of the opening:

Going Home After Gastropexy Surgery

Your dog had a laparoscopic gastropexy, which is a preventive surgery that attaches the stomach to the inside wall of the belly. Golden Retrievers are at higher risk for a serious condition called GDV, or "bloat and twist," where the stomach flips over on itself. This surgery prevents that from happening. You made a smart choice by having it done before anything went wrong.

The full document continues with sections on incision appearance, medication instructions with practical dosing guidance, e-collar rationale (with warmth about why it matters), activity restrictions, feeding guidance, a day-by-day description of what normal recovery looks like, specific warning signs that require a call, and follow-up appointment details.

Step 4: your review.

Three things to adjust.

The gabapentin explanation says "helps with pain and also with the anxiety that often comes with surgery recovery." Not wrong, but you prescribe gabapentin primarily for pain in this case, and the anxiety framing could confuse the owner into thinking you're treating their dog for anxiety. Change to: "This is for pain management during the first five days of recovery. Give it on schedule, not only when your dog seems uncomfortable."

Add a line at the end of the warning signs section: "Call us with any questions. We would rather hear from you with a 'probably fine' question than miss something that wasn't fine." That single sentence changes how anxious owners behave at 11pm when they're worried.

The clinic contact information placeholder needs your actual clinic phone and the after-hours emergency number. Add those before printing.

Step 5: what went home.

A document with seven clear section headers, plain-language explanations, and enough specific detail that the owner can refer back to it at 11pm if they're worried. Total time to produce: about six minutes. Old way, written from scratch or modified from a generic template: fifteen to twenty minutes, and the result is usually less warm than this.

The owner goes home with a document that anticipates the questions they'll actually have. They call the clinic less. They feel cared for. Their dog recovers without incident. Nobody takes a photo of this discharge document for social media, but this is exactly the kind of small, compounding improvement that distinguishes a practice over time.

Building Your Handout Library

After you've used AI to generate discharge instructions for a condition a few times and refined the output to match your practice's voice and clinical standards, save that document. Name it clearly. Keep a folder, in Google

Drive, on your desktop, wherever is convenient, organized by condition or procedure type.

Within a few months of regular use, you'll have a library of polished, reviewed, practice-specific handouts for 20 or 30 common presentations. New staff can use them. You can update them when protocols change. You never start from scratch on a routine discharge document again.

That library compounds in value over time in a way that individual AI interactions do not. Build it deliberately.

Chapter 6

Client Communication - The Hard Conversations and the Routine Ones

If you have been practicing for more than a year, you already know that the technical skills of veterinary medicine (the surgery, the diagnostics, the pharmacology) aren't actually the hardest part of the job.

The hardest part is the communication.

It is explaining to the Ramírez family that their 11-year-old golden retriever has osteosarcoma and that the most realistic outcome, even with aggressive treatment, is measured in months. It is calling back the client who left a one-star review because they felt dismissed when they came in for their cat's third urinary episode in six months. It is writing to the referring cardiologist about the cat you just found that has late-stage mitral valve disease, in language professional enough to be taken seriously and clear enough to transfer the clinical picture accurately.

These aren't documentation tasks. They're relationship tasks that require writing. And that distinction matters, because AI is a writing tool, not a relationship tool.

What that means in practice: AI cannot tell you what to say to the Ramirez family. But it can give you a first draft of the letter that helps you say it, so that when you sit down to write that conversation at 8pm after a hard day, you're editing and personalizing rather than staring at a blank page wondering where to start.

This chapter covers the full range of client communication: from the clinical letter to the difficult conversation to the online review response. For each one, we will establish the limits first, and then show you where AI genuinely helps.

Diagnosis and Clinical Update Letters

Whenever a patient is referred, when test results come back after an appointment, or when a diagnosis carries implications for long-term management, a clear, well-written letter to the client matters. These letters become part of the relationship. A family who receives a thoughtful, personalized letter explaining their dog's Cushing's diagnosis and what to expect going forward feels cared for. A family who gets a printout of a lab report with no context does not.

AI drafts these letters well. The key is giving it the clinical details plus the emotional context.

The clinical letter prompt:

"Write a letter from a veterinarian to a pet owner. The tone should be warm, clear, and empathetic. This is a relationship communication, not a form letter. The owner is knowledgeable about their pet but does not have a medical background.

Patient: [De-identified signalment]

Diagnosis: [Plain language]

What this means for the pet: [Day to day impact, prognosis if appropriate]

Treatment plan: [What the owner needs to do and why]

What to watch for at home: [Signs of progression or complication]

Follow-up plan: [What happens next]

The tone for this specific letter should be: [Warm and reassuring / Direct and informative / Compassionate and realistic]"

That last line, specifying the tone, is very important. A letter delivering a manageable chronic diagnosis calls for a different register than a letter following a terminal diagnosis conversation. Tell the tool what you need.

The Letters Nobody Wants to Write

Some client letters are harder than others. Not harder to draft. Harder to sit down and start. The cancer diagnosis. The end-of-life conversation follow-up. The letter to a family after a patient did not survive an emergency.

AI can help you start these. Not by writing the emotional content for you. That has to come from you, because it's about your patient and your relationship with that family. But by giving you a structural framework and a first draft that you then make your own.

A few principles for using AI on these letters:

Give the tool the clinical facts and the emotional context. "The family had this dog for 14 years and were shocked by the diagnosis" gives the tool something to work with in terms of tone.

Read the draft as a starting point, not a finished product. These letters need your voice. Edit them significantly. Add the specific detail that only you know: the thing the client mentioned in the exam room, the name of the dog they lost five years ago, the moment during the appointment that mattered to them.

Never send an AI-generated draft of a difficult letter without reading it thoroughly.

Here is a prompt for a terminal diagnosis follow-up letter:

"Write a follow-up letter from a veterinarian to a pet owner after a terminal diagnosis conversation. The tone should be deeply compassionate, honest, and warm. This is not a form letter. It should feel personal. Avoid clinical coldness and avoid false optimism. Acknowledge the difficulty of what the family is facing while offering clarity and support.

Patient: [De-identified signalment]

Diagnosis: [What was found and what it means]

What was discussed in the appointment: [Key points covered]

What the family's options are: [Briefly: comfort care, palliative, or specific treatment if applicable]

What the family should expect in terms of timeline: [If known and appropriate to include]

What support you are offering: [Availability for questions, referral to oncology, etc.]

What the next step is: [Who reaches out, when, about what]"

Responding to Negative Online Reviews

This section is uncomfortable for most clinicians because the instinct when someone criticizes your work online is either to defend yourself or to ignore it entirely. Neither is the right move.

A thoughtful, professional, non-defensive response to a negative review does more for your reputation than the absence of a response, and it often does more for the reviewer relationship as well. The person who left a one-star review because they felt rushed is sometimes a client who can be recovered. Even when they can't, other prospective clients read your response.

Before we get to the prompt, a hard limit: do not discuss clinical details in a public online response. Do not reference the patient's condition, the treatment, the medications, or anything about the clinical encounter in a public forum. Client confidentiality applies. Keep public responses general, empathetic, and focused on the relationship, not the medicine.

Here is a framework for a negative review response:

Acknowledge the experience without agreeing with the characterization.

Express genuine concern that they felt that way.

Invite them to contact you directly to discuss.

Keep it to two or three sentences.

The prompt:

"Write a professional, empathetic response to a negative online review from a veterinary client. The response should acknowledge their experience without admitting fault or making clinical claims, express that their concern matters, and invite direct contact. Keep it to 2-3 sentences. Do not be defensive. Do not mention any clinical details.

The review expressed the following concern: [Summarize the concern in general terms - e.g., 'the client felt they were rushed and not listened to during the appointment']"

Review the output carefully. Edit it to sound like you, not like a corporate response template. The goal is genuine, not polished.

Here is what a good AI-assisted response looks like after your review and light editing:

"Thank you for taking the time to share your experience. We are sorry your visit did not meet the standard we hold ourselves to, because every client deserves a clear explanation and time to ask questions. We would genuinely like to hear more about what happened and make it right. Please reach out to us directly at [phone number] so we can speak with you personally. We appreciate your feedback and hope to have the opportunity to do better."

That took two minutes to generate and thirty seconds to review. It's professional, it's human, and it doesn't escalate. That is the goal.

Multilingual Client Communication

The reality of modern veterinary practice is that not all of your clients speak English as their first language. A discharge instruction written in clinical English that a client can't fully understand isn't actually a discharge instruction. It's a piece of paper they took home and couldn't use.

AI tools can translate client-facing documents into Spanish, Mandarin, Portuguese, Vietnamese, and many other languages with reasonable accuracy.

This is one of the more powerful and underused applications in veterinary practice.

A few cautions. For clinical documents, always have a bilingual staff member or colleague review AI-translated text before it goes to a client. Translation errors in a medication instruction or a warning sign can cause real harm. For non-clinical communication such as welcome letters, appointment reminders, or general practice information, the risk is lower and AI translation is often excellent.

The workflow: write the English version first, review it for accuracy and clarity, then ask the AI tool to translate it into the target language with a note that it's a veterinary client education document and should use plain language appropriate for a non-medical reader. Then, and this is important, have someone fluent in that language review the translation if at all possible before you use it as a clinic standard. AI translation is good. It is not perfect. For a document that will be used repeatedly with patients, a one-time human review is worth the effort.

For one-off situations such as a client who needs an explanation of today's diagnosis in Spanish and you don't have a staff member who can help, AI translation is a reasonable bridge. Be transparent with the client that this is a translation aid, not a professionally certified document. Most clients appreciate the effort.

The prompt structure for translated documents:

"Translate the following veterinary client handout into [language]. Keep the tone warm and clear. Flag any medical terms that may not translate directly and offer a plain-language explanation in the target language.

[Paste your English document here]"

Vaccine and Wellness Reminders

Routine client communication, including vaccination reminders, annual wellness recall notices, and follow-up reminders for patients whose recommended rechecks were never scheduled, is exactly the kind of writing that should take almost no time. It isn't complex. It doesn't require clinical nuance. It just needs to be warm, clear, and specific enough to motivate action.

Build a set of reminder templates for your core reminder types: annual wellness, dental month, heartworm prevention season, senior wellness, and post-visit follow-ups. Generate each one with AI, review and refine it once, and use it repeatedly.

AI handles this in seconds. Give it the context: the patient, the overdue service, the tone of your practice. Then ask for a short, friendly reminder message appropriate for email or text. Save it as a template and adapt it for each scenario.

A prompt that works:

"Write a short, friendly email reminder for a dog owner whose pet is overdue for annual vaccines and a heartworm test. The practice name is [your practice name]. Warm tone, not pushy. Include a clear call to action to call or book online. Under 100 words."

Build a small library of these: annual wellness, rabies overdue, dental recheck, post-diagnosis follow-up that was never scheduled. Once the templates exist, sending them is a staff function. You are out of the loop entirely.

Financial Conversations and Estimate Follow-Ups

Nobody enjoys the financial conversation. Veterinary care is expensive, clients are often unprepared for what a workup costs, and the gap between what you can do and what they can afford is one of the genuine ethical weights of this work. These conversations happen in the room, and sometimes they need to happen in writing, in a follow-up email that summarizes the estimate, explains the options, and gives the client time to make a decision without the pressure of the exam room.

Written financial communication needs to be clear, non-judgmental, and structured around the client's ability to make an informed decision. It should present the options honestly, note the clinical implications of each path, and make clear that you're there to help them navigate whatever they decide.

AI can draft these well. The key is giving it the full range of options you discussed, not just the ideal treatment plan, but the stepped-down options and the monitoring-only option if that's clinically appropriate, and asking it to present each with the same respect and without editorializing.

Then review it carefully. These letters touch on clinical prognosis, financial specifics, and sometimes implicit or explicit decisions about an animal's welfare. Read every line. Make sure it accurately reflects what you said in the room and what you're comfortable putting in writing.

Treatment estimate summary letter:

"Write a brief letter to accompany a treatment estimate for a pet owner. The tone is warm and non-pressuring. Explain the recommended treatment, why it is recommended, and what it involves. Briefly acknowledge that this is a significant cost and that the team is available to discuss options. Do not be apologetic about the cost of care. Frame it as information the owner needs to make the best decision for their pet.

Treatment recommended: [Description in plain language]

Why it is recommended: [Brief clinical rationale in plain language]

Estimated cost: [Add after AI generates the document]

Alternative options if applicable: [Any tiered options being offered]

Contact for questions: [Your clinic name -- add after]"

Follow-up after a client declines recommended treatment:

This is a difficult letter to write, and it matters clinically and legally. When a client declines a recommended treatment, documenting that the recommendation was made and that the client was informed of the risks of declining is part of the clinical record. A brief, non-judgmental follow-up letter also keeps the door open for a client who may reconsider.

"Write a brief, non-judgmental follow-up letter to a pet owner who declined the recommended treatment during their visit. Acknowledge that they heard the recommendation. Restate the core concern in plain language. One sentence. Note that the clinic is available if they have questions or if they would like to reconsider. The tone should be warm and supportive, not guilt-inducing. No medical jargon.

The condition discussed: [Plain language description]

The recommendation that was declined: [Brief description]

The key risk of not treating: [One sentence, plain language]

What they should watch for at home: [Specific signs that should prompt a return]"

That letter, reviewed and sent, serves both the relationship and the clinical record. Keep a copy in the patient file.

Case Study: A Difficult Letter, And What the AI Invented

This is the hardest kind of client communication, and it's where AI-assisted drafting earns its place most clearly. You need to write well. You're not in a state to write well at 8pm after a day that included a terminal diagnosis conversation. AI bridges that gap, with one serious caveat that this case study is designed to show.

The setup: a twelve-year-old female spayed Labrador, metastatic pulmonary cancer diagnosed three days ago, owner is a retired veterinarian who understands the diagnosis completely. She cried during the in-clinic conversation. You agreed on comfort care. She asked for a follow-up letter.

You give the AI your clinical bullet points and the right prompt framing, including the emotional context and the tone you want. Warm, honest, not clinical. What comes back is a two-page letter that's close to ready, with real warmth in it. Good draft, fast. That is the value proposition.

Now the caveat.

Somewhere in the middle paragraph, the AI's draft reads: "Bella has been your companion for twelve years."

You didn't put a name in your clinical notes. The AI invented it.

This is a hallucination, and in a condolence letter it's potentially a relationship-ending error. If that letter had gone out with a fabricated dog name, the client would have noticed immediately. A retired veterinarian reading a letter about her dying dog would register the wrong name as either carelessness on your part or, worse, evidence that the letter wasn't really from you at all.

The rule from Chapter 1 applies here in its most important form: every AI output must be read carefully before anything goes out. In clinical documentation, the thing to catch is usually a drug dose or a clinical detail. In relationship communication, the thing to catch can be a fabricated personal detail that sounds entirely natural in context.

The workflow that works: give the AI good clinical and emotional context, let it draft, then read every sentence twice. Change what needs changing. Replace what's wrong. Add the specific personal details the AI couldn't know. The version that goes to the client should be a letter the AI could not have written alone, because it contains things only you could have added.

Total time, start to finish: about eight minutes for a letter that would have taken you thirty minutes from a blank page at the end of a hard day. The value is real. So is the responsibility to read every word.

Making AI Sound Like Your Practice

This is the piece most people skip and then wonder why their AI-assisted communication feels generic.

Every practice has a voice. Some are formal and clinical: white-coat professional, precise language, minimal warmth. Some are warm and familiar, they know your dog's name and your kids' names and they remember that your cat hates the carrier. Most are somewhere in between, and that voice is part of what clients are choosing when they choose your practice.

AI defaults to a neutral, moderately professional tone that doesn't belong to anyone in particular. Left uncorrected, that tone makes your client communication sound like it came from a veterinary chain's corporate office rather than from the people who have been caring for their animals for years.

The fix is simple: tell the AI what your voice sounds like before you ask it to write. You can do this in a short paragraph at the top of any prompt.

"Our practice tone is warm and informal. We use first names, we avoid medical jargon, we are direct but never cold. We want clients to feel like they are hearing from a friend who happens to be a veterinarian, not from a business."

Or: "Our practice is professional and precise. We use proper medical terminology when it is appropriate, explain it when we use it, and maintain a respectful, caring tone. We are not informal but we are never clinical to the point of coldness."

Write that description once. Save it. Paste it at the top of every client communication prompt. The output will sound like your practice from the first draft.

You can also train the tool on your existing writing. Paste in two or three examples of client emails you have written and liked, the ones that felt right, and ask the tool to match that style. "Here are three examples of how I write to clients. Match this tone and style in the letter I am about to ask you to write." That instruction, combined with good examples, produces output that is much closer to your actual voice.

The full range of client communication, from the routine wellness reminder to the letter that follows a terminal diagnosis, is where your practice's relationship with its clients either deepens or erodes. AI doesn't replace the judgment, the empathy, or the clinical knowledge that makes that communication meaningful. But it removes the friction that prevents it from happening well. It gives you a draft when you're tired. It gives you language when you're searching for words. It gives you a starting point that would have taken twenty minutes to reach on your own.

Used well, it makes your communication better, not because AI writes better than you, but because you communicate better when you're not exhausted by a blank page.

That is worth something. In a profession with the burnout rates veterinary medicine carries, anything that removes friction and returns mental energy to the work that actually matters is worth quite a bit.

Chapter 7

Running Your Practice - Operations and Staff

Running a veterinary practice means doing two jobs at once. The clinical job is the one you trained for. The operational job is the one that fills the hours nobody planned for: the hiring, the policies, the staff communication, the compliance documentation.

The clinical job gets most of the attention. The operational job gets most of the hours.

Hiring, onboarding, training, scheduling, compliance documentation, staff policies, performance conversations, team meetings. None of it is why you went to veterinary school. But it's a substantial portion of what running a practice actually requires. And it generates an enormous volume of writing. Job postings. Training materials. SOPs. Memos. Policy documents. Performance notes. None of it is clinical. All of it takes time.

AI handles operational writing well. It doesn't require clinical judgment, which means the verification burden is lower. It doesn't require deep specificity about an individual patient, which means the privacy considerations are simpler. What it requires is clear context about your practice, your team, and what you need the document to do. Give it that, and it will give you a solid first draft in minutes.

This chapter covers the operational writing your practice generates and where AI fits into each category. It also covers where it does not fit, because managing a team involves judgment, relationship, and legal nuance that no writing tool can substitute for.

Standard Operating Procedures

SOPs are among the highest-value documents in a veterinary practice, and among the most neglected. Most practices acknowledge the importance of SOPs in principle, but few maintain comprehensive, current documentation across all clinical and operational areas. The AAHA accreditation process specifically calls out SOP gaps as a common finding. And DEA audit data is striking: an AAHA estimate suggests that approximately 96% of practices would fail a DEA inspection due to recordkeeping errors that clear SOPs would prevent.

The problem isn't that practice owners don't understand the value of SOPs. The problem is that writing them from scratch is time-consuming, and in a practice where clinical work fills every hour, operational documentation gets deferred indefinitely.

AI removes the drafting barrier. You bring the process knowledge. The tool turns it into a document.

The prompt for an SOP:

"Write a standard operating procedure for a veterinary practice. The SOP should be clear enough that a new employee could follow it without additional guidance. Use numbered steps. Include the purpose of the procedure, who is responsible, the steps in order, and any safety or compliance notes.

Procedure: [Describe the process in plain terms, e.g., 'how we receive, log, and store controlled substance shipments']

Practice context: [Any specifics, e.g., 'small animal general practice, 3 DVMs, 2 exam rooms, VetStar PIMS']"

Review the output carefully. SOPs for controlled substances, anesthesia, and any regulated process must be reviewed against current DEA and state board requirements before use. AI will produce a well-structured document. Compliance is your responsibility to verify.

Areas where SOP drafting is high-value: controlled substance receiving and logging, patient check-in and check-out workflow, anesthesia setup and monitoring, surgical suite prep and breakdown, inventory management, after-hours emergency protocols, equipment maintenance and log requirements, and infection control procedures.

Staff Onboarding Materials

Onboarding new team members takes time that most practices don't have. Research cited by VetPartners shows that 68% of employees prefer learning through structured materials, and practices with clear onboarding processes see lower turnover in the critical first 90 days. Yet most practices hand a new hire a stack of policies and a working schedule and call it onboarding.

AI can help you build the materials that make onboarding structured without requiring someone to sit down and write a manual from scratch.

Useful onboarding documents that AI drafts well: welcome letters that explain practice culture and expectations, role-specific orientation checklists, practice tour guides describing what is where and who to ask about what,

FAQ documents for new hires, and summaries of key policies in plain readable language.

The prompt for an onboarding welcome letter:

"Write a welcome letter from a veterinary practice to a new employee. The tone should be warm and welcoming while setting clear expectations. The letter should cover: what the first week will look like, who they will be working with, what they should know about our culture and values, and how to get help if they have questions. Practice context: [Brief description of your practice: size, type, focus]. New employee role: [Position]."

Review for accuracy and add the personal touch that makes a welcome letter feel genuine rather than generated.

Training Materials and CE Documentation

New protocols, equipment rollouts, updated compliance requirements: your team needs to be trained on these, and documentation of that training matters for regulatory purposes. AI drafts training materials that are structured, clear, and digestible.

"Write a one-page training guide for veterinary staff on [topic]. The audience is [role, e.g., veterinary technicians]. The guide should cover: why this matters, the key steps, common mistakes to avoid, and what to do if something goes wrong. Keep the language clear and practical."

AI is also useful for creating the quiz or assessment questions that document training completion. Straightforward, verifiable, and something no one wants to spend time writing from scratch.

Job Postings and Hiring Communications

Hiring is one of the most time-consuming operational challenges in veterinary practice. The 2024 AVMA Report on the Economic State of the Veterinary Profession cited staff recruitment and retention as the top operational concern for independent practices. Writing a job posting that accurately reflects the role, appeals to qualified candidates, and stands out in a competitive market is harder than it looks.

AI drafts job postings quickly and can be directed to emphasize whatever matters most to your practice: culture, schedule, compensation structure, growth opportunity.

"Write a job posting for a [position] at a veterinary practice. Emphasize: [what matters most, e.g., a collaborative team culture, opportunities for skill development, work-life balance, or specific clinical skills]. Practice type: [Description]. Requirements: [Key qualifications]. Compensation: [Add after AI drafts]."

AI also drafts offer letters, rejection emails, and interview confirmation messages: the administrative correspondence around hiring that takes real time to write individually.

Policy Documents

Employee handbooks, PTO policies, code of conduct expectations, social media policies, a practice AI use policy. These are documents that practices need, tend not to have in writing, and defer writing because the blank page is daunting.

For a policy document prompt:

"Draft a [policy name] for a veterinary practice. The policy should be clear, professional, and fair. Cover: the purpose of the policy, who it applies to, the specific rules or expectations, and the consequences for violation. Practice context: [Brief description]."

One important note: employment policies have legal implications that vary by state. Before implementing any policy document, have it reviewed by an employment attorney or your practice management consultant. AI will draft a solid starting point. The legal review is not optional.

Internal Communication

Staff memos, team announcements, schedule changes, policy reminders: the day-to-day internal communication of a busy practice is low-glamour and time-consuming. AI handles it in seconds.

"Write a staff memo announcing [topic, e.g., a new scheduling system, a policy change, a team celebration]. The tone should be [professional and direct / warm and positive / matter-of-fact]. The memo should include: what is changing, when it takes effect, what staff need to do, and who to contact with questions."

Keep AI-generated memos short, personalize them before sending, and make sure they sound like you, not like a corporate communication template.

Staff Meeting Agendas and Minutes

A well-structured agenda helps a meeting stay on track. A clear set of minutes ensures decisions are documented and action items are followed up on. Both take time to write. Neither requires clinical judgment.

"Write a staff meeting agenda for a veterinary practice. The meeting is [duration] and covers the following topics: [List topics]. Format it so each item includes the topic, who is presenting, and how much time is allocated."

For minutes: "Write meeting minutes based on the following notes from our staff meeting. The minutes should be clear, professional, and capture decisions made and action items assigned. Notes: [Paste your raw notes]."

Performance Documentation

Performance documentation is one of the most important and most avoided parts of practice management. When a personnel issue eventually requires formal action, the quality of the documentation trail matters enormously , and that matters legally and practically.

AI can help you draft performance improvement plans, formal written warnings, and documentation of verbal counseling sessions. The key is giving it accurate factual input and reviewing the output carefully.

"Draft a performance documentation memo for an employee. The memo should be professional, factual, and specific. It should describe: what was observed or reported, the date and context, what the expectation is, and what the next step will be if the behavior continues. Do not editorialize. Stick to observable facts. Employee role: [Role]. Issue: [Factual description]."

Two hard limits here. First: AI cannot make personnel decisions for you. Who to hire, who to counsel, who to let go: those are your decisions, made with your knowledge of the whole person and the whole situation. AI can help you document those decisions clearly. It cannot make them. Second: anything that involves termination, discrimination concerns, or potential legal exposure should involve your employment attorney. A well-written

AI-generated document does not substitute for legal counsel when the stakes are high.

What AI Cannot Do in Practice Operations

AI writes documents. It does not manage people.

The hardest parts of running a practice team are the parts that happen in conversation: the direct feedback that a team member's performance is not meeting expectations, the conflict between two staff members that has been building for months, the exit interview with someone who is leaving because they feel undervalued. These require human presence, relationship, and judgment. They cannot be delegated to a writing tool.

Use AI to prepare for those conversations: to draft talking points, to organize your thoughts, to ensure the documentation that follows is clear and accurate. Do not use it as a substitute for having them.

Prompt Library - Practice Operations

Staff onboarding checklist:

"Write an onboarding checklist for a new [role] at a veterinary practice. Include: paperwork and HR steps, equipment and system access, orientation tasks for the first day, week, and month, and key people to meet. Format as a checklist."

Practice social media policy:

"Draft a social media policy for a veterinary practice team. Cover: acceptable and unacceptable posts involving the practice, patients, or colleagues; patient privacy obligations; consequences for violations; and who to contact with questions."

Emergency protocol summary:

"Write a one-page emergency protocol summary for veterinary practice staff. Cover: who to call in an after-hours emergency, how to handle client calls requesting emergency care, and what to document."

Staff recognition communication:

"Write a brief all-staff message recognizing [employee or team] for [specific accomplishment]. The tone should be warm and genuine, not corporate. Keep it to three or four sentences."

New equipment rollout memo:

"Write a staff memo announcing that we are implementing [new equipment or system]. Cover: what it is, why we are implementing it, when training will happen, and what staff need to do to prepare."

Scheduling change notification:

"Write a brief, professional message to staff notifying them of [schedule change]. Be direct and clear. Include the effective date, what is changing, and who to contact with questions."

Chapter 8

Exotics, Large Animals, and the Edge Cases

Here's something you need to know before you use AI for anything outside of dogs and cats: the tools you're working with were trained on data. A lot of data. And the distribution of that data matters enormously.

The veterinary literature, the online forums, the case reports, the textbooks, the clinical notes that were digitized and incorporated into AI training datasets, and they're overwhelmingly about companion animals. Dogs and cats represent the vast majority of documented clinical experience in the data these tools learned from. A 2025 review in the American Journal of Veterinary Research was explicit about this: species diversity is a distinct challenge for veterinary AI, because physiological differences across species require species-specific training data that simply doesn't exist at scale for most non-canine and non-feline animals.

What that means practically: an AI tool used to write clinical documentation for a rabbit, a bird, a bearded dragon, or a horse will do so with the same confidence it uses for a Labrador with a UTI. The output will look professional. The drug names will be spelled correctly. The format will be right. And the clinical content may be significantly wrong.

This chapter is about understanding where that risk lives and how to work around it.

The Confidence Problem

The most important thing to understand about AI output on non-canine and non-feline species is that AI does not know what it does not know.

When you ask an AI tool to draft a discharge instruction for a rabbit with GI stasis, it won't pause and say its training data on lagomorphs is limited. It will generate a document. That document will sound like every other discharge instruction it has seen. And it may contain drug recommendations, dosages, or monitoring instructions that are appropriate for a different species or that reflect outdated practice.

This is not a flaw unique to exotic animal documentation. You saw it in Chapter 4 with feline patients. Cats metabolize drugs differently than dogs, and AI handles those differences inconsistently. With exotics, the problem is amplified because the underlying data is thinner. There's simply less published veterinary documentation about rabbits, birds, reptiles, ferrets, and guinea pigs in the sources these tools were trained on, relative to the clinical complexity and species-specific nuance involved.

The rule for exotics and large animals: use AI for the writing and the structure. Apply your own clinical expertise to every clinical detail. That division of labor, AI handling the drafting and you handling the medicine, applies throughout this book, but it's especially important here.

Exotic Companion Animals

Rabbits, guinea pigs, ferrets, chinchillas, and rats are common enough in general practice that most DVMs see them regularly. They're also species where the gap between confident AI output and accurate clinical content is genuinely dangerous.

Rabbits are obligate herbivores with a GI physiology entirely unlike companion carnivores. Drug sensitivities in rabbits are well-documented and serious. Penicillin and amoxicillin, for example, are contraindicated in rabbits due to fatal enterotoxemia risk, yet these are drugs an AI tool might suggest for a respiratory case if it draws on canine and feline respiratory treatment patterns. NSAID use in rabbits requires specific caution around renal function. Anesthesia protocols differ significantly from small animals and carry higher risk.

Guinea pigs cannot synthesize vitamin C, which has implications for wound healing and immune function that are clinically relevant and unlikely to be reflected accurately in AI-generated output. Ferrets have a high incidence of adrenal disease and insulinoma that requires specific monitoring and documentation considerations. Chinchillas are highly sensitive to heat stress and have dental disease patterns that are genuinely different from other small mammals.

None of this is obscure. Any veterinarian who sees exotics knows it. The point is that AI does not know it reliably, and its output will not warn you when it is wrong.

How to use AI with exotic companion animals: use it to draft the structural elements of your documentation. The format of the SOAP note, the organization of the discharge instruction, the structure of the client handout. Then fill in every clinical detail yourself. Do not let an AI-generated drug name, dose, or monitoring recommendation leave your practice without independent verification against a current exotic formulary or specialist reference.

The prompt approach that works: provide explicit clinical parameters in your prompt to reduce hallucination risk. Rather than "write a discharge instruction for a rabbit with GI stasis," try: "Write the structure of a discharge instruction for a rabbit patient with GI stasis. Leave all medication names, doses, and specific clinical instructions as [FILL IN] placeholders that I will complete. I will provide the clinical content." That approach gets you the formatting and the client-language structure without risking incorrect clinical content making it into the final document.

Avian Patients

Birds present a distinct documentation challenge because normal physiological parameters, drug metabolism, and clinical signs differ not just from mammals but substantially across avian species. The difference between a budgerigar and a macaw is not just size. It involves different nutritional requirements, different drug sensitivities, different normal ranges, and different behavioral and clinical presentations of illness.

AI's training data on birds is thin relative to companion animals, and it isn't uniformly distributed across avian species. Output about psittacines may be somewhat more reliable than output about raptors, softbills, or poultry, simply because there's more published clinical material on companion parrots. But even for common companion birds, the confidence-accuracy gap is real.

For avian clients, the translation layer matters enormously. Avian owners are often deeply attached and highly informed. A discharge instruction that uses approximations or inaccurate clinical language will be noticed. AI can help you write warm, clear, organized client communication. It cannot reliably supply the avian-specific clinical content.

Avian-specific documentation considerations: always verify drug dosages against a current avian formulary such as the Exotic Animal Formulary or avian specialist references. Normal temperature ranges, heart rate, and respiratory rate differ significantly from mammals and should be provided explicitly in your prompts rather than left for AI to fill in. Nutritional instructions for avian patients require species-level specificity that AI will not provide reliably.

Reptiles and Amphibians

Reptiles and amphibians represent the thinnest end of AI's training data in veterinary medicine. The published clinical literature is smaller, the species diversity is enormous, and the physiological differences from mammals are fundamental.

Temperature-dependent metabolism means that environmental management is central to clinical care in a way that has no parallel in mammalian medicine. A bearded dragon's response to medication depends partly on its body temperature. A tortoise in hibernation has a completely different metabolic state than one in active season. An AI tool drafting clinical documentation for a reptile will not incorporate these realities accurately, because the training data doesn't support it.

This doesn't mean AI is useless for reptile and amphibian documentation. It means the division of labor is even more important. Use AI to produce the structural scaffold: the organization of the SOAP note, the headings of the client handout, the format of the discharge document. Supply all clinical content yourself. Every drug name, every dose, every environmental requirement, every monitoring instruction. Do not let AI fill in clinical gaps for reptile and amphibian cases.

One area where AI is genuinely helpful for reptile and amphibian clients: translating complex husbandry requirements into plain language. If you need to explain UVB lighting requirements, appropriate temperature gradients, or humidity management to a first-time reptile owner, AI can take your clinical knowledge and turn it into a readable, organized handout in less than two minutes. That application, AI as a language translator rather than a clinical source, is where it adds real value.

Equine and Large Animal

Equine and large animal practice presents different challenges from exotics, but the underlying issue is the same: AI was trained predominantly on small animal companion medicine, and its output on equine, bovine, ovine, and caprine cases should be treated with additional scrutiny.

Normal vital signs for horses differ substantially from companion animals. Drug dosages are weight-dependent in ways that require careful calculation. Controlled substance protocols in equine practice involve specific considerations around DEA compliance that may not be reflected accurately in AI output. Common equine conditions such as colic, laminitis, respiratory disease, and lameness have clinical nuance and treatment protocols that require verification against current equine references.

There's also an operational dimension unique to large animal and equine practice. Many large animal veterinarians are ambulatory, practicing in field conditions, at farms, at competition venues, without consistent internet connectivity. Documentation often happens after the fact, from notes or voice memos captured during the appointment. AI is genuinely useful for this workflow: paste in your field notes and get a structured, professional record in return. But the connectivity constraint means having a reliable mobile workflow, and the clinical verification step is non-negotiable.

The ambulatory documentation workflow: capture your clinical notes immediately after the appointment, while the case is fresh. Voice memo on your phone works well in field conditions. When you have connectivity, de-identify and paste those notes into your AI tool with a clear prompt specifying the species, the normal ranges you observed, and the clinical parameters. Use the output as a structural draft. Verify all drug names, doses, and clinical recommendations before finalizing.

For equine and large animal practitioners, purpose-built platforms are beginning to address the historically thin tool landscape. Products like CoVet have introduced equine-specific templates developed with equine practitioners, and platforms like StableTrack are designed specifically for equine practice management workflows. These tools may outperform general-purpose AI for equine documentation because they're trained on more relevant clinical data. Appendix C has a current overview of tools available in this space.

Building Your Own Species-Specific Context

One of the most effective techniques for improving AI output on non-standard species is building a context block: a paragraph of species-specific clinical information that you paste at the top of every prompt for that species. Think of it as briefing the tool before you put it to work.

A context block for rabbit patients might look like this:

"The following involves a rabbit patient. Key species context for documentation: Rabbits are obligate herbivores and hindgut fermenters. They are highly sensitive to antibiotics that alter gut flora, including penicillins, cephalosporins, and lincosamides. NSAID use requires renal monitoring. Normal temperature 101-104 F, heart rate 130-325 bpm, respiratory rate 30-60 breaths per minute. GI motility is critical and must be maintained.

Do not suggest any medications or treatments that are not specified in my clinical notes."

A context block for avian patients might include the species name, normal ranges for that species, and an explicit instruction not to fill in clinical content not provided in your notes.

Build these context blocks once for the species you see regularly. Save them. Paste them at the top of every prompt for that species. The output will be more structurally useful and less likely to contain plausible-sounding but clinically incorrect content.

The Edge Cases

Beyond the major categories above, general practice occasionally encounters species that fall entirely outside what any AI tool can be expected to handle reliably: sugar gliders, hedgehogs, prairie dogs, injured wildlife, zoo animals referred for specialist care. For these cases, the rule is simple: use AI only for the structural and client-communication elements, treat every clinical detail as something that requires your expert input, and do not mistake confident-sounding output for accurate output.

The more unusual the species, the thinner the training data, and the greater the risk. That is not a reason to avoid AI for documentation. Documentation of unusual cases takes real time, and AI can help organize and structure that documentation. It is a reason to be more deliberate about the division of labor, not less.

A Note on Client Communication Across Species

One application of AI that works consistently well regardless of species is client communication that doesn't involve clinical specifics. Welcome letters to new exotic pet owners that describe your practice's approach to exotic animal care. Educational handouts about general husbandry principles that you then fill in with species-specific details. Follow-up emails that check in on a patient after a procedure, with the specific clinical monitoring instructions provided by you rather than generated by AI.

Clients who own non-traditional pets are often highly engaged and deeply invested in their animals. Good client communication matters to them. AI helps you produce it faster and more consistently, as long as you're the one supplying the clinical content.

Prompt Library - Exotics and Large Animals

Species-specific SOAP note structure:

"Write the structural skeleton of a veterinary SOAP note for a [species] patient. Leave all clinical details as [FILL IN] placeholders. Include the appropriate section headers and indicate within each section what type of information belongs there, without generating specific clinical content. I will complete all the clinical details myself."

Exotic patient client handout structure:

"Write the structure of a client education handout for a [species] patient being treated for [condition described in general terms]. Leave all medication names, doses, monitoring values, and specific clinical instructions as [FILL IN] placeholders. Format the handout with clear sections and plain language for a non-medical reader."

Husbandry translation:

"Translate the following husbandry requirements into plain, clear language for a first-time [species] owner. Focus on the practical: what they need to do, in what order, and what to watch for. My clinical notes on required husbandry: [Paste your notes]."

Field notes to structured record:

"I am a large animal veterinarian. The following are rough field notes from a farm call today. Convert these into a structured veterinary record with appropriate SOAP format sections. Do not add clinical details not present in my notes. Species: [Species]. Notes: [Paste de-identified field notes]."

Referral letter for exotic patient:

"Write the structure of a referral letter for a [species] patient being referred to an exotic animal specialist. Leave clinical details as [FILL IN] placeholders. The letter should include sections for patient signalment, reason for referral, history summary, findings to date, diagnostics performed, and current status."

Chapter 9

Staying Current - AI as a Learning Tool

Veterinary medicine moves fast. New drug approvals, updated treatment protocols, emerging resistance patterns, changing regulatory requirements, guideline revisions from the AVMA and specialty colleges: the volume of new information a practicing veterinarian is expected to absorb and integrate is genuinely relentless. And the continuing education system, while valuable, addresses only a fraction of it. Thirty hours of CE every two years covers the requirement. It does not cover the field.

Most veterinarians stay current through a combination of habit and hustle: scanning journal abstracts, following professional listservs, attending conferences when the schedule allows, relying on colleagues for the informal knowledge transfer that happens when practitioners compare notes. It works, mostly. But it's also fragmented, time-inefficient, and heavily dependent on what you happen to encounter rather than what you actually need.

AI does not replace any of that. What it does is compress the time between encountering a question and getting a useful orienting answer, and it does that consistently, on demand, at 11pm after a difficult day when no colleague is available and no conference is scheduled.

This chapter is about using AI as a learning tool: to explore clinical questions, prepare for CE, orient yourself on unfamiliar topics, and stay current more efficiently. It also covers where that use has hard limits, because in medicine, the source of information matters as much as the information itself.

AI as a Starting Point, Not a Finishing Point

The most important frame for this chapter is also the simplest one: AI is a starting point for learning, not a finishing point.

When you ask an AI tool a clinical question, about a drug interaction, an emerging treatment protocol, a condition you rarely see, you're getting a synthesis of the text the tool was trained on, weighted toward what was most common and most frequently represented in that training data. You're not getting a citation, a peer-reviewed finding, or a current guideline. You're getting a well-organized summary of what the AI learned from a large body of text, with a cutoff date, and with all the limitations of the training data that informed it.

That is genuinely useful as an orienting step. It is not sufficient as a clinical conclusion.

Think of it the way you would think of talking through a case with a well-read colleague who has not seen the most recent literature. They can help you think through the landscape, remind you of considerations you might have overlooked, and point you toward the right questions. But you still check the current guidelines, verify the dosage in a current reference, and apply your own clinical judgment to the specific patient in front of you.

Used that way, AI accelerates learning without replacing the rigor that clinical medicine requires.

Exploring Clinical Questions

One of the most natural uses of AI in a clinical setting is the quick orienting question: what do I know about this, and what should I be thinking about?

A patient presents with a condition you see infrequently. You have a working diagnosis, a treatment plan forming, and a few minutes before your next appointment. You can type a quick prompt and get a structured summary of the current thinking on that condition: its presentation, common differentials, typical treatment approaches, monitoring considerations. You review it with your clinical eye. You note anything that prompts a follow-up in a more authoritative source. You go see the next patient.

That interaction isn't replacing your training or your judgment. It is functioning like a very fast, very organized refresher that surfaces what you already know and flags what you might want to verify.

A prompt structure that works for clinical orientation:

"Summarize the current understanding of [condition] in [species]. Include: typical presentation, common differentials, standard treatment approaches, and any monitoring considerations I should keep in mind. I am a practicing DVM, not a student. Give me a clinical-level summary, not a basic introduction."

That last instruction matters. Without it, AI tools tend to pitch clinical content at a general audience. Specifying that you're a practicing clinician usually shifts the response to a more appropriate register.

Two cautions. First: drug dosages from AI should always be verified against a current formulary before use. The tool may not have the most current recommendations, and species-specific dosing in particular warrants independent verification. Second: for conditions where current guidelines are actively evolving, including emerging infectious diseases, recently updated treatment protocols, new drug approvals: AI's training cutoff means the information may be outdated. Check the primary source.

Using AI to Prepare for CE

Continuing education is more useful when you arrive with context. Walking into a two-hour session on a topic you haven't thought about in three years is a different experience than walking in with a working understanding of the landscape and specific questions you want answered.

AI can compress the orientation step dramatically. Before a CE session or conference presentation on a topic:

"I am attending a CE session on [topic] for veterinary practitioners. Give me a one-page overview of the current landscape: the key concepts I should already know, the questions the field is currently debating, and what has changed in the past two years. I want to walk in with context, not starting from scratch."

That prompt typically produces a genuinely useful briefing document. Review it critically and apply the same caution about recent developments that you would apply to any AI-generated clinical content. As a way of walking into a learning session better prepared, it's one of the highest-value applications in this chapter.

You can also use AI after a CE session to consolidate and apply what you learned:

"I just attended a continuing education session on [topic]. Here are the key points I took away: [your notes]. Help me think through how to apply these in my practice. What follow-up questions should I be researching? Are there any implementation considerations I should think about?"

That kind of consolidation prompt turns passive attendance into active integration.

Reading and Understanding Research

Keeping up with the veterinary literature is genuinely difficult when you're seeing patients eight hours a day. Journals publish continuously. Most abstracts are opaque to anyone who isn't already immersed in the specific subfield. And the gap between what is published and what is clinically applicable is often significant.

AI can help bridge some of that gap, with an important caveat: do not paste copyrighted journal content into public AI tools. That applies both to privacy considerations and to copyright obligations. What you can do:

Paste an abstract (abstracts are typically accessible and publicly available) and ask for help interpreting it: "Here is the abstract from a veterinary research paper. Explain what this study found, its key limitations, and whether its findings are likely to be applicable in general small animal practice. Be direct about where the evidence is strong and where it is not: [Paste abstract]."

Ask for context around a finding you encountered: "A continuing education speaker mentioned [specific finding or claim]. Can you help me understand the evidence base for this and whether it represents current consensus or an emerging or contested position?"

Ask for orientation on a research area you want to explore: "I want to get more current on the literature around [topic] in veterinary medicine. What are the key research questions being actively studied, and what would be the most useful journals or types of publications to follow?"

None of these replace reading the literature. They reduce the friction that prevents you from engaging with it in the first place.

Building a Personal Learning System

The veterinarians who use AI most effectively for learning tend to have a consistent habit, not an occasional one. They ask questions as they arise during the day rather than batching them into a learning session that never quite happens. They treat AI interactions as the first step of a two-step process: AI for orientation, primary sources for verification and depth.

A practical framework:

Capture questions as they arise. Keep a running note on your phone, in your PIMS, wherever you capture things, of clinical questions, unfamiliar conditions, drug interactions you were uncertain about, and topics you want to understand better. These are your learning agenda. Do not let them evaporate at the end of a busy day.

Batch the AI step. At some natural break, lunch, end of day, whenever you have ten minutes, run your captured questions through an AI tool. Get orienting answers. Flag what needs verification against a primary source. Flag what's clearly in your knowledge base and can be dismissed.

Verify the important ones. Clinical questions that will actually affect patient care go to a primary source: Plumb's for drug questions, current AVMA or specialty college guidelines for protocol questions, peer-reviewed literature for emerging evidence questions. AI gives you the map. Primary sources give you the territory.

Keep a personal reference file. When you find a high-quality answer to a question you expect to encounter again, document it. The verified answer, with the source. Over time this builds a personal reference library that reflects your specific practice and patient population.

What AI Gets Wrong in Clinical Learning

Understanding the failure modes matters as much as understanding the value.

AI is confidently wrong about dosages with some regularity, particularly for less common species and less common drugs. The output sounds exactly like correct information. Always verify.

AI's training data has a cutoff. For topics where the field has moved meaningfully in the past one to two years, including new drug approvals and updated treatment guidelines, emerging resistance patterns, recent guideline revisions: the AI may reflect the old consensus rather than the current one. Ask it when it thinks the information was last current, and treat recent topics with extra skepticism.

AI reflects the distribution of its training data, which means common conditions and common species are better represented than rare conditions and uncommon species. Its depth on canine parvovirus is not the same as its depth on ferret adrenal disease. Calibrate your confidence accordingly.

AI can synthesize confidently from limited or contradictory sources. In areas where the evidence is genuinely thin or actively debated, AI may produce a summary that sounds more settled than the actual state of the literature. Ask it directly: "Is there genuine consensus on this, or is this a contested or evolving area?"

None of these limitations make AI useless for learning. They make it necessary to use it with the same critical eye you would apply to any source that's useful but imperfect.

AI as a CE Topic in Itself

One specific application of AI as a learning tool deserves its own mention: using it to understand AI.

The tools are changing rapidly. New capabilities, new limitations, new applications in veterinary practice. The AVMA is actively developing guidance. State boards are beginning to address disclosure and appropriate use. The landscape is genuinely evolving, and staying current on the tool itself is part of using it responsibly.

The AAHA has introduced CE programming specifically on AI in veterinary medicine. The AVMA's Task Force on Emerging Technologies is producing resources on appropriate use. These are worth engaging with, not just to understand what's coming, but to be a participant in shaping how the profession adopts these tools rather than a passive recipient of decisions made elsewhere.

Chapter 10
The Road Ahead

This book has stayed deliberately close to the ground. Practical workflows. Specific prompts. Clear limits. Applications you can use tomorrow, in your actual practice, with the patients you actually see.

This chapter looks up from the immediate and says: here's where this is going. Not as prediction, because predicting the pace and direction of AI development has proven to be a reliable way to be wrong, but as orientation. The decisions you make now about how to integrate AI into your practice won't be made in a vacuum. They will be made in the context of a field that is moving, and understanding the direction of that movement helps you make better decisions today.

Where Things Stand Now

In 2025 and 2026, the most widespread applications of AI in veterinary practice are exactly what this book has covered: documentation assistance, client communication, practice operations. These are the applications that are accessible, affordable, and immediately useful. They require no special equipment, no system integration, and no waiting for regulatory clarity. They work now.

Alongside these, a second category of tools is moving from pilot projects into practical use in larger and specialty practices: AI-assisted diagnostic imaging interpretation. Roughly two dozen companies now market AI software for veterinary radiograph review, and the technology is expanding into cytology and pathology interpretation. The American College of Veterinary Radiology and the European College of Veterinary Diagnostic Imaging published a joint position statement in 2025 establishing guiding principles for the ethical development and use of these tools, acknowledging both their transformative potential and the continuing necessity of expert human interpretation. The technology is real, it is in use, and it is improving.

A third category is earlier in the adoption curve but moving quickly: ambient documentation tools. These are AI systems that listen to exam room conversations and generate structured clinical notes automatically, without the veterinarian typing or dictating. Products like CoVet and HappyDoc are in active use in practices across the country, with practitioners reporting meaningful reductions in documentation time and end-of-day chart burden. The ambient documentation category is likely to become the dominant form of AI-assisted documentation in veterinary practice within the next several years, as the technology matures and workflow integrations with major PIMS platforms become standard.

What Is Coming

A 2025 panel at the AVMA Veterinary Business and Economic Forum featured Dr. Petra Harms, John J. Craig, PhD of MetronMind, and Dr. Jeremy Redmond of Louisiana State University. The panel described a clinic where AI quietly manages background tasks, triaging patients, drafting records, generating cost estimates, and streamlining communication, while veterinarians focus on diagnosis, surgery, prescribing, and the human work of empathy and relationship. As Dr. Craig put it: the goal is not to replace the human element but to automate the boring parts so veterinarians can spend their time on care and communication.

Researchers at Cornell have demonstrated AI tools capable of predicting whether cats have intestinal inflammation or lymphoma from ultrasound image analysis. Researchers elsewhere are using AI to predict chronic kidney disease in cats from health record data two years before clinical signs emerge. Predictive models for herd health in livestock operations are flagging illness before clinical signs develop. AI systems embedded directly in digital radiography units classify and orient images as soon as they're captured.

None of this is science fiction. All of it is happening in research settings and, increasingly, in clinical practice.

What it adds up to is a profession in transition. The veterinarians who will be most effective in ten years are not the ones who resisted these tools or the ones who adopted them uncritically. They're the ones who developed clear thinking about where AI adds value, where it requires human oversight, and where human judgment is irreplaceable, and who built their practices and their clinical habits accordingly.

What Does Not Change

As AI capabilities expand, some things remain constant. They're worth naming explicitly, because the pace of change can make it easy to lose sight of them.

Your clinical judgment is irreplaceable. AI can help you draft documentation faster, interpret imaging more efficiently, and manage your practice more effectively. It cannot examine a patient. It cannot read the room in a difficult conversation with a grieving family. It cannot make the judgment call that distinguishes a patient who needs emergency care from one who can safely wait. The veterinarian at the center of every patient encounter is not a historical artifact. It is the foundation of what veterinary medicine is.

The VCPR is yours. Chapter 1 established this and it bears repeating here. No AI tool, however capable, can hold the veterinarian-client-patient relationship. No AI tool can assume clinical responsibility. The veterinarian is and must remain the accountable party in every patient encounter. The expanding capabilities of AI tools don't change this, and the AVMA Task Force on Emerging Technologies has been explicit about it.

Your professional obligations do not change with the tools. Privacy obligations apply regardless of which tools you use. Disclosure obligations are evolving, but the underlying ethic of transparency with clients doesn't change. The standard of care is still defined by what a competent veterinarian would do in similar circumstances, and the tools you use are part of how you meet or fail to meet that standard.

The relationship with your clients is still the foundation. Clients choose veterinary practices for the quality of their animals' care, the trust they have in the clinician, and the relationship they have built over years of appointments. AI can make you more efficient, more consistent, and better at the written communication that supports that relationship. It cannot build the relationship. That work remains yours.

How to Stay Oriented as Things Change

The landscape is moving fast enough that specific tools and specific capabilities will change by the time this book is in its second printing. What stays stable is the framework for evaluating any new tool.

Ask what it does, specifically. When a vendor or a colleague describes an AI tool, ask what it actually does: what data does it use, what does it produce, what has it been validated on, who has reviewed that validation? Vague claims about AI-powered capabilities deserve specific questions.

Ask where the human oversight sits. For any AI application in a clinical setting, there should be a clear answer to the question: where does the trained professional review and validate this output? If the answer is that the tool handles it, that's a red flag. If the answer is that the tool produces a draft and the clinician approves it before it affects care, that's the appropriate model.

Ask about the evidence. For tools making clinical claims such as diagnostic support, treatment recommendations, and risk prediction, ask what the validation evidence looks like. Is it peer-reviewed? Is it published? Is it specific to the species and conditions in your practice? The absence of premarket regulatory requirements for veterinary AI tools means the burden of evaluation falls on the practitioner. That is not comfortable, but it is the current reality.

Stay connected to professional guidance. The AVMA, AAHA, specialty colleges, and state boards are all actively developing guidance on AI use in veterinary practice. This guidance will evolve, and staying current with it is part of practicing responsibly with these tools. The profession is in the process of establishing its own norms, and practitioners who engage with that process help shape it.

Chapter 11

Your Prompt Library - Copy, Paste, and Go

This chapter is a working reference. Every prompt here is ready to copy directly into any major AI tool (ChatGPT, Claude, Gemini, or Grok) with your de-identified clinical details filled in where indicated by brackets.

A few reminders before you start. De-identify before you paste: remove client names, patient names, addresses, and any detail that could identify a specific animal or owner. Review every output before it's used: read it with your clinical eye, verify drug names and doses against a current reference, and correct anything that's wrong. These prompts get you to a strong first draft in seconds. Your review is what makes it clinical documentation.

The prompts are organized by category. Use the section headings to find what you need during your actual workday.

Troubleshooting: When AI Does Not Do What You Expected

Every practicing clinician who uses these tools regularly runs into the same handful of frustrations. Here's how to recognize and fix each one.

The AI gives you a generic, stiff output that sounds like no one you know.

The most common cause is a thin prompt. "Write a SOAP note for a dog with vomiting" will get you a generic SOAP note. "Write a SOAP note for a 7-year-old male neutered Labrador Retriever presenting for vomiting x3 days with the following clinical findings..." will get you something useful.

The second cause is no tone guidance. AI defaults to a neutral, vaguely professional register. If you want warm, say warm. If you want direct and clinical, say so. One line at the top of any client-facing prompt ("Our practice is warm and conversational. Avoid medical jargon. Write like you are speaking to a friend who happens to be worried about their pet.") transforms the output.

The AI invents a fact that wasn't in your notes.

This is hallucination, and it happens most often in two situations: when your input leaves clinical gaps, and when you ask for something the AI cannot verify.

The fix is to add an explicit instruction at the end of every clinical prompt: "Do not add clinical details, medications, doses, or findings that are not specifically provided in my notes. If a section is incomplete, leave it incomplete and flag it rather than filling it in."

You will still need to read every output carefully. But that instruction reduces the rate of invented details significantly.

The AI refuses to help with a legitimate clinical task.

This happens occasionally with consumer AI tools when the subject involves controlled substances, euthanasia, or certain drug combinations. The tool is being cautious in ways that don't fit clinical context.

Two ways to get through it. First, add context at the top of your prompt: "I am a licensed veterinarian drafting clinical documentation for a real patient in my care. This is not a public-facing document." Second, if that fails, reframe the task away from the trigger word. Instead of asking for help "drafting a euthanasia consent form," ask for help "drafting an end-of-life care authorization document." Same content, different wrapper, usually works.

If neither works, that tool may not be the right one for that task. Try a different AI tool or handle that document manually.

The AI's output is close to right but awkwardly worded.

You don't need to start over. Ask for specific edits. "Rewrite this paragraph in a warmer tone." "Shorten the introduction by half." "Restate this using plain language a non-medical reader can follow." "Remove the clinical abbreviations and spell everything out."

Iterating is faster than regenerating from scratch, and the tool retains the context of what it already produced.

The AI flags uncertainty you don't think is warranted.

Some tools are trained to hedge more than is necessary. If you know the correct answer and the AI hedged, edit the output to the correct answer. The AI is not a colleague you need to negotiate with. It is a draft tool. You are the clinician. Overwrite.

The AI won't tell you that it doesn't know something.

This is the opposite problem, and it's more dangerous. Consumer AI tools rarely say "I do not know" outright. They produce a confident-sounding answer even when the information is outside their training data.

The safeguard is your review. Every drug name verified. Every dose checked against a current formulary. Every clinical claim read for accuracy. If something in an AI-generated output feels too specific to be general knowledge, it probably came from somewhere specific, and you should verify it before trusting it.

The tool is slow or unavailable at the moment you need it.

Consumer AI tools have peak usage hours. Late afternoon and early evening on weekdays are often slower than early mornings or late nights. If you're consistently running into speed problems during your actual workday, the paid tier of your chosen tool will usually solve it. Twenty dollars a month, and you get faster responses and priority access.

You realize you pasted identifying information into the AI by mistake.

This is a more serious situation than it may first appear, and the correct response is not to panic but also not to dismiss it.

First, do not immediately delete the conversation. You will need to know exactly what was disclosed in order to understand your obligations. Screenshot it or make a written record of what information was in the prompt before you take any other action.

Second, understand that this may have regulatory and professional implications depending on your state. Most state veterinary practice acts impose confidentiality obligations on client and patient information, and all fifty states plus DC have data breach notification laws that can apply when personal information is disclosed to an unauthorized third party. Whether an accidental disclosure to a consumer AI tool triggers a specific reporting requirement depends on your state, what information was disclosed, and the AI tool's data handling practices. There's no universal answer.

Third, contact your state veterinary medical board for guidance and consider consulting an attorney familiar with professional licensing and state privacy law. Most boards would rather hear about an accidental disclosure from you with a question about next steps than discover it later through a client complaint. Calling early is almost always better than calling late.

Fourth, once you understand your obligations, follow them. This may include notifying the affected client, depending on what was disclosed and what your state requires. Client notification, when required, is almost always better received when you initiate it than when the client finds out another way.

Fifth, delete the conversation from the AI tool and review whether its privacy settings were configured appropriately for clinical use. Most consumer AI tools let you delete conversations, which removes them from your account history. How long the data is retained on the tool's servers, and whether it was used to train future models, depends on the tool's privacy policy and the settings you had enabled.

Sixth, and most important going forward: make the de-identification step non-negotiable in your workflow. If you find yourself tempted to skip it "just this once," that's the moment to pause. The ten seconds is always worth it.

This book cannot tell you what your specific state requires, and nothing in this section is legal advice. That is exactly why Chapter 1 asked you to build an AI use policy for your practice before you start using these tools. A policy that anticipates how your practice will handle accidental disclosure means you'll know what to do before it happens, instead of improvising under pressure.

SOAP Notes and Clinical Documentation

General SOAP Note - Full Draft

"You are helping a veterinarian document a patient visit. Write a complete SOAP note using the clinical information below. Use professional veterinary language. Be specific about all medications including generic names, doses in mg/kg where relevant, total doses, routes, and frequency. Do not add clinical details that are not provided. Flag any section where you are uncertain rather than guessing.

[Paste de-identified clinical notes]"

Subjective Section Only

"Write the Subjective section of a veterinary SOAP note based on the following owner-reported history and chief complaint. Capture the key clinical history in professional language. Patient is [signalment].

[Paste de-identified owner history and chief complaint]"

Plan Section - Clinician Use

"Write the Plan section of a veterinary SOAP note for the following case. Include all medications with doses, routes, and frequency. Include diagnostics ordered, follow-up timing, and client instructions provided. Use professional veterinary clinical language. Do not add clinical details that are not provided.

[Paste de-identified plan details]"

Plan Section - Technician Handoff Format

"Write the Plan section of a veterinary SOAP note formatted as a clear technician task list. Organize by task order. Include all medications with doses, routes, and frequency. Be specific enough that a veterinary technician can execute the plan without asking for clarification.

[Paste de-identified plan details]"

Recheck / Progress Note

"This is a recheck visit. Write the Subjective section as a progress note. The patient was previously treated for [condition] with the following plan: [brief prior plan summary]. Today the owner reports the following: [de-identified owner update]. Patient is [signalment]."

Multi-Problem Case

"Write the Assessment and Plan sections of a SOAP note for a patient with multiple active problems. Address each problem separately with its own Assessment and Plan, clearly labeled. Patient is [signalment].

Problem 1: [Description and relevant findings]

Problem 2: [Description and relevant findings]

Problem 3: [Description and relevant findings]"

Referral Letter

"Write a professional referral letter from a general practice veterinarian to a specialist. The letter should summarize the patient's history, clinical findings, diagnostics performed, current working diagnosis, treatments attempted, and the reason for referral. Use professional veterinary language. Be thorough.

Patient signalment: [De-identified signalment]

Reason for referral: [Specialty and specific reason]

History: [De-identified history]

Clinical findings: [De-identified exam findings]

Diagnostics performed and results: [De-identified results]

Working diagnosis: [Your clinical assessment]

Treatments attempted: [What you have tried]"

Lab Result Follow-Up Note

"Write a brief clinical note documenting a telephone follow-up with a client regarding laboratory results. Include what was discussed, what the results mean, what the client was instructed to do, and any follow-up plan.

Patient signalment: [De-identified signalment]

Results discussed: [De-identified results]

Clinical significance: [Your interpretation]

Client instructions given: [What you told the client]

Follow-up plan: [Next steps]"

Surgical Report Narrative

"Write the narrative portion of a surgical report for a veterinary procedure. Include a description of the procedure, significant intraoperative findings, any complications, and the immediate recovery period. Do not add findings not provided.

Procedure: [Procedure name and description]

Intraoperative findings: [De-identified findings]

Complications: [None / Description]

Recovery: [Patient status at end of procedure]"

Discharge Instructions

Core Discharge Prompt

"Write discharge instructions for a pet owner. Use warm, clear, non-medical language. Avoid clinical abbreviations. Organize with clear section headers. Patient is [signalment: species, breed, age, sex].

Diagnosis / reason for visit: [Plain language description]

Treatment provided today: [What was done]

Medications going home: [Drug name, dose in practical terms, frequency, duration, purpose -- one line per medication]

Activity restrictions: [Specific restrictions and duration]

Diet: [If applicable]

Wound/incision care: [If applicable]

Warning signs to watch for and when to call: [List specific signs]

Follow-up: [When and why]

Clinic contact: [Add after AI generates]"

Post-Surgical Discharge

"Write detailed post-surgical discharge instructions for a pet owner. Warm, clear, plain language. Patient is [signalment].

Procedure performed: [Plain language description]

What was found: [If applicable]

Incision location and current appearance: [Describe]

Pain medication going home: [Name, dose, frequency, duration]

Other medications: [List if applicable]

E-collar: [Yes/no, how long, why]

Activity restrictions: [Specific and time-bound]

What normal healing looks like over the next 10 days: [Key milestones]

Warning signs that require a call: [List specific signs]

Suture removal / recheck: [When and what will happen]"

Post-Spay / Neuter

"Write discharge instructions for a pet owner after their [dog/cat] was spayed/neutered today. Patient is [signalment]. Anesthesia was uneventful. E-collar provided. Home with [pain medication name, dose, frequency, duration]. Activity restriction: [duration]. Suture removal in [X] days. Warning signs: incision opening, swelling, excessive licking, lethargy beyond 24 hours, not eating beyond 24 hours, discharge from incision site."

Acute Gastroenteritis

"Write discharge instructions for the owner of a [dog/cat] seen for vomiting and/or diarrhea. Patient is [signalment]. [Diagnosis in plain language]. Medications going home: [list with practical doses and frequency]. Dietary instructions: [bland diet, how long, how to transition back]. Warning signs to call: vomiting more than twice in 24 hours, blood in stool or vomit, lethargy, not improving after 48 hours."

Urinary Tract Infection

"Write discharge instructions for the owner of a [dog/cat] diagnosed with a urinary tract infection. Patient is [signalment]. Antibiotic going home: [name, dose in practical terms, frequency, duration]. Importance of completing the full course. Signs of improvement to watch for. Signs that it is not improving: still straining, blood in urine after 5 days, lethargy, not eating. Recheck urinalysis at [timeframe]."

Chronic Disease Home Care Guide

"Write a comprehensive home care guide for a pet owner whose [dog/cat] has been diagnosed with [condition]. The owner is motivated but has no medical background. Cover: what [condition] is and what causes it, how it affects the pet day-to-day, the treatment plan [list medications and monitoring], how to monitor at home, what to do if they miss a dose, dietary requirements, exercise guidelines, follow-up schedule, and questions to bring to the next appointment. Tone: warm and empowering."

Client Communication

Diagnosis / Clinical Update Letter

"Write a letter from a veterinarian to a pet owner. Warm, clear, empathetic. This is a relationship communication, not a form letter. The owner is knowledgeable about their pet but does not have a medical background.

Patient: [De-identified signalment]

Diagnosis: [Plain language]

What this means for the pet: [Day-to-day impact, prognosis if appropriate]

Treatment plan: [What the owner needs to do and why]

What to watch for at home: [Signs of progression or complication]

Follow-up plan: [What happens next]

Tone for this specific letter: [Warm and reassuring / Direct and informative / Compassionate and realistic]"

Terminal Diagnosis Follow-Up Letter

"Write a follow-up letter from a veterinarian to a pet owner after a terminal diagnosis conversation. Deeply compassionate, honest, and warm. Not a form letter -- it should feel personal. Avoid clinical coldness and avoid false optimism.

Patient: [De-identified signalment]

Diagnosis: [What was found and what it means]

What was discussed in the appointment: [Key points covered]

What the family's options are: [Comfort care, palliative, or specific treatment if applicable]

What support you are offering: [Availability for questions, referral, etc.]

What the next step is: [Who reaches out, when, about what]"

Negative Online Review Response

"Write a professional, empathetic response to a negative online review from a veterinary client. Acknowledge their experience without admitting fault or making clinical claims. Express that their concern matters and invite direct contact. 2-3 sentences. Not defensive. No clinical details.

The review expressed the following concern: [Summarize in general terms]"

Wellness Reminder

"Write a short, friendly email reminder for a [dog/cat] owner whose pet is overdue for [wellness visit / specific vaccine / dental exam]. Practice name: [your practice name]. Warm tone, not pushy. Brief line about why this care matters. Clear call to action to schedule. Under 100 words."

Estimate Accompanying Letter

"Write a brief letter to accompany a treatment estimate for a pet owner. Warm and non-pressuring. Explain the recommended treatment, why it is recommended, and what it involves. Acknowledge the significant cost and that the team is available to discuss options. Do not be apologetic about the cost of care. Frame it as information the owner needs to make the best decision for their pet.

Treatment recommended: [Description in plain language]

Why it is recommended: [Brief clinical rationale in plain language]

Alternative options if applicable: [Any tiered options being offered]

Contact for questions: [Your clinic name -- add after]"

Declined Treatment Follow-Up

"Write a brief, non-judgmental follow-up letter to a pet owner who declined the recommended treatment. Acknowledge they heard the recommendation. Restate the core concern in one plain-language sentence. Note the clinic is available if they have questions or reconsider. Warm, supportive tone. No medical jargon.

The condition discussed: [Plain language description]

The recommendation that was declined: [Brief description]

The key risk of not treating: [One sentence, plain language]

What they should watch for at home: [Specific signs that should prompt a return]"

Multilingual Translation

"Translate the following veterinary client handout into [language]. Keep the tone warm and clear. Flag any medical terms that may not translate directly and offer a plain-language explanation in the target language.

[Paste your English document here]"

Practice Operations and Staff

Standard Operating Procedure

"Write a standard operating procedure for a veterinary practice. Clear enough that a new employee could follow it without additional guidance. Use numbered steps. Include the purpose, who is responsible, the steps in order, and any safety or compliance notes.

Procedure: [Describe the process]

Practice context: [Brief description of your practice]"

Staff Onboarding Welcome Letter

"Write a welcome letter from a veterinary practice to a new employee. Warm, welcoming, and clear. Cover: what the first week will look like, who they will be working with, what they should know about our culture and values, and how to get help. Practice context: [Brief description]. New employee role: [Position]."

Onboarding Checklist

"Write an onboarding checklist for a new [role] at a veterinary practice. Include: paperwork and HR steps, equipment and system access, orientation tasks for day one, week one, and month one, and key people to meet. Format as a checklist."

Staff Training Guide

"Write a one-page training guide for veterinary staff on [topic]. Audience: [role]. Cover: why this matters, the key steps, common mistakes to avoid, and what to do if something goes wrong. Clear and practical language."

Job Posting

"Write a job posting for a [position] at a veterinary practice. Emphasize: [what matters most]. Practice type: [Description]. Requirements: [Key qualifications]. Compensation: [Add after AI drafts]."

Performance Documentation Memo

"Draft a performance documentation memo for an employee. Professional, factual, and specific. Describe: what was observed or reported, the date and context, what the expectation is, and what the next step will be if the behavior continues. Do not editorialize. Stick to observable facts. Employee role: [Role]. Issue: [Factual description]."

Staff Memo

"Write a staff memo announcing [topic]. Tone: [professional and direct / warm and positive]. Include: what is changing, when it takes effect, what staff need to do, and who to contact with questions."

Controlled Substance Compliance Policy

"Write a controlled substance compliance policy for a veterinary practice. Cover: which staff are authorized to handle controlled substances, logging requirements for each transaction, storage security requirements, reconciliation procedures, and what to do if a discrepancy is found. Practice context: [Brief description]."

Exotics and Large Animals

Species-Specific SOAP Structure

"Write the structural skeleton of a veterinary SOAP note for a [species] patient. Leave all clinical details as [FILL IN] placeholders. Include appropriate section headers and indicate what type of information belongs in each section. I will complete all clinical details myself."

Exotic Patient Discharge Structure

"Write the structure of a client education handout for a [species] patient being treated for [condition described in general terms]. Leave all medication names, doses, monitoring values, and specific clinical instructions as [FILL IN] placeholders. Clear sections, plain language for a non-medical reader."

Husbandry Translation

"Translate the following husbandry requirements into plain, clear language for a first-time [species] owner. Focus on the practical: what they need to do, in what order, and what to watch for. My clinical notes on required husbandry: [Paste your notes]."

Field Notes to Structured Record

"I am a large animal veterinarian. The following are rough field notes from a farm call today. Convert these into a structured veterinary record with appropriate SOAP format sections. Do not add clinical details not present in my notes. Species: [Species]. Notes: [Paste de-identified field notes]."

Exotic Referral Letter Structure

"Write the structure of a referral letter for a [species] patient being referred to an exotic animal specialist. Leave clinical details as [FILL IN] placeholders. Include sections for patient signalment, reason for referral, history summary, findings to date, diagnostics performed, and current status."

Continuing Education and Learning

Clinical Orientation

"Summarize the current understanding of [condition] in [species]. Include: typical presentation, common differentials, standard treatment approaches, and any monitoring considerations I should keep in mind. I am a practicing DVM. Give me a clinical-level summary, not a basic introduction."

CE Preparation Briefing

"I am attending a CE session on [topic] for veterinary practitioners. Give me a one-page overview of the current landscape: the key concepts I should already know, the questions the field is currently debating, and what has changed in the past two years."

CE Consolidation

"I just attended a CE session on [topic]. Here are the key points I took away: [your notes]. Help me think through how to apply these in my practice. What follow-up questions should I be researching?"

Abstract Interpretation

"Here is the abstract from a veterinary research paper. Explain what this study found, its key limitations, and whether its findings are likely to be applicable in general small animal practice. Be direct about where the evidence is strong and where it is not.

[Paste abstract]"

Chapter 12

Your 30-Day Launch Plan

You've read the book. You know the principles, the limits, the workflows, and the prompts. Now the question is: where do you start?

This chapter is a structured 30-day plan that takes you from first use to AI as a working part of your daily practice. It's designed for someone starting from zero. If you're already using some of these tools, treat it as a guide to expanding and systematizing what you've already started.

The plan is built around one core insight: consistency matters more than intensity. You don't need to use AI for every task on day one. You need to use it regularly enough that the workflow becomes habit. Habit is what makes the time savings compound. A tool you use three times a week every week is worth far more than a tool you use twenty times in a burst and then set aside.

Thirty minutes a week is enough to make meaningful progress. One new workflow per week is the right pace.

Before You Begin

Before day one, complete three things.

Fill in your AI policy. Appendix D has a template. It takes fifteen minutes. Having it written down, specifically what you will use AI for, what you will never use it for, and what your review process is, means you aren't making these decisions under the time pressure of a busy clinic day.

Open an account on your chosen tool. ChatGPT, Claude, Gemini, or Grok. Free tier is fine to start. If you don't have an account, create one before day one. The learning curve starts with the first interaction.

Read the de-identification workflow in Appendix B. Make it a habit before you develop any other habit. It takes ten seconds and it protects your clients. Do it automatically from your first day.

Week One: SOAP Notes

The highest-return starting point. You write SOAP notes every day. The time savings are immediate and cumulative.

Day 1: Run the walkthrough from Chapter 3. Use the practice scenario in that chapter. This is a dry run with no real patient data. Get a feel for how the tool responds and how prompting works before you use it on a real case.

Days 2-3: Use AI for one real SOAP note. Choose a straightforward case: a wellness visit, a routine illness presentation, nothing complex. De-identify your notes, paste them in with the general SOAP note prompt from Chapter 11, and review the output carefully.

Days 4-5: Try the Subjective-only and Plan-only prompts on two different cases. Notice which sections AI handles best and where your review catches errors.

Days 6-7: Use AI for three to five SOAP notes across the week. Track how long the review takes. You should be getting comfortable with the workflow by the end of the week.

One discipline for the whole week: every AI-generated SOAP note gets reviewed before it goes in the record. No exceptions. Build the habit now.

Week Two: Discharge Instructions

The second highest-return application. Discharge instructions take meaningful time to write well and AI handles them consistently.

Days 8-9: Use the Core Discharge Prompt on two cases from your normal workload. Compare the output to what you would have written. Notice where AI gets the structure right and where the clinical specifics need your hand.

Days 10-11: Try the Post-Surgical Discharge prompt if you do surgical work. If not, use the Chronic Disease Home Care Guide prompt for a patient you're currently managing.

Days 12-13: Use the condition-specific prompts, UTI, gastroenteritis, dental, or whichever is most relevant to your practice, and save the best output as a template.

Day 14: You should have at least three to five discharge instruction templates by end of week two. Name them clearly and store them where you can find them. This is the beginning of your handout library.

Week Three: Client Communication

Letters, reminders, estimate letters, difficult follow-ups.

Days 15-16: Write one clinical update or diagnosis letter using the prompts from Chapter 6. Choose a case where the client needs written follow-up. Review carefully, because these go directly to clients and need to sound like you, not like a generic template.

Days 17-18: Generate three reminder templates: one for annual wellness, one for dental, one for a condition-specific recall relevant to your practice. These will be used by staff, so review them with your front desk in mind.

Days 19-20: Use AI to draft an estimate accompanying letter for a case with a significant treatment recommendation. Review it carefully before sending.

Day 21: If you have a negative review that has been sitting without a response, draft a response this week. If not, write a template response for a common type of concern and have it ready.

Week Four: Operations and Expansion

Practice operations and building out your system.

Days 22-23: Identify the one SOP your practice most needs that doesn't currently exist in writing. Use the SOP prompt to draft it. Review it, correct it to match your actual workflow, and circulate it to your team.

Days 24-25: If you have a hiring need, draft a job posting. If not, draft an onboarding checklist for one role in your practice. Either way, you're building operational documentation that will save time in the future.

Days 26-27: Use AI for one CE preparation briefing before a webinar, journal article, or other learning activity you've scheduled this month.

Day 28: Review what you've built over the past four weeks. Count your templates. Identify the two or three workflows that saved you the most time. These are your core use cases, the ones to protect and refine going forward.

Day 29: Decide what to add next. Chapter 6 has the client communication prompts. Chapter 7 has the operations prompts. Chapter 8 has the exotics and large animal prompts. Chapter 9 has the learning prompts. Identify one area you haven't yet used and plan for it in month two.

Day 30: Update your AI policy if anything has changed based on experience. Note any cases where AI output needed significant correction. These are signals about where to apply extra scrutiny. Note the places where the output was excellent with minimal review. Those are your most reliable use cases.

After 30 Days

By the end of the first month, you should have a working set of SOAP note prompts you trust, a library of discharge instruction templates, at least a few client communication templates, and some operational documentation you didn't have before.

More importantly, you should have a feel for where AI earns its keep and where it needs your eye most carefully. That knowledge is specific to your practice, your patient population, and your own documentation style. No book can give it to you. Thirty days of consistent use can.

The compounding starts now. Every template you save, every prompt you refine, every workflow you systematize: these accrue. A year from now, the library you've built will be one of the more useful assets in your practice.

The paperwork was never the point. This is about getting it out of the way so you can do the work that actually matters. You became a veterinarian to take care of animals. The tools are finally good enough to help you do that.

Chapter 13

Documentation Compliance Quick Reference

This appendix is a condensed reference for the documentation requirements that govern veterinary practice in the United States. It is designed to sit at your desk or be printed and posted. It is not legal advice. Requirements vary by state and change over time. Always verify current requirements with your state veterinary medical board and, for controlled substances, with the DEA.

Medical Records: What Belongs in Every Patient File

The AVMA and AAHA establish the baseline standard. Most state veterinary practice acts require the following at minimum.

Patient identification

Species, breed, age, sex, reproductive status, owner name and contact information, and a unique patient identifier.

Date and attending veterinarian

Date of each visit, with the name or initials of the attending veterinarian.

Chief complaint and history

What the owner reported, in enough detail that another clinician could reconstruct the clinical context.

Physical examination findings

Vital signs, weight, body condition score, and system-by-system examination results. "Normal" is an acceptable finding when documented explicitly. "WNL" without specifics is not.

Assessment

Your working diagnosis or differential list, with clinical rationale. This section is the legal record of your professional judgment. It must reflect what you actually concluded, not a generic category.

Plan

Every medication prescribed or administered (name, strength, dose, route, frequency, duration, lot number for controlled substances), diagnostics ordered, referrals made, client education provided, and follow-up schedule.

Consent documentation

Signed informed consent for anesthesia, surgery, euthanasia, and any procedure carrying material risk. Document verbal consent when written consent isn't obtained, including the date and context.

Client communication log

Telephone calls, email follow-ups, and in-clinic conversations that involve clinical decisions. Include advice given, advice declined, and the client's response.

Dispensing record

For any medication sent home: drug name, strength, quantity dispensed, lot number, expiration date, and client instructions.

Records should be legible, organized, and complete enough that a colleague, a relief veterinarian, or a licensing board investigator can understand the case from the documentation alone. The AVMA standard: if it wasn't documented, it didn't happen.

Controlled Substance Logs: Federal Requirements

Under the Controlled Substances Act (21 U.S.C. Section 821) and DEA regulations, any veterinary practice registered to dispense or administer Schedule II through V controlled substances must maintain the following.

Separate log per schedule

A separate dispensing log for each schedule. Combined logs across schedules do not meet the requirement.

Required fields per entry

Date, patient name and species, drug name and strength, quantity administered or dispensed, dose given, route of administration, running balance remaining in clinic stock, and the name or initials of the authorized person who administered or dispensed.

Reconciliation

Entries must reconcile exactly with patient records and with physical inventory.

Retention

DEA minimum: two years from the date of the transaction. Many states require three to five years. Check your state requirement and apply the longer of the two.

Authorized personnel only

Controlled substance logs must be signed by a DEA-registered veterinarian or authorized designee.

Discrepancies

A running balance that does not match physical inventory, or a log entry with no corresponding patient record, triggers formal reporting obligations. Do not attempt to correct or back-fill discrepancies without legal guidance.

AI has no role in the actual log entries. Policy documents, training materials, and audit preparation checklists are appropriate AI applications. The log itself is a human-only document with a required chain of accountability.

Record Retention: Minimum Periods by Category

General patient records

Most states require three to five years from the last contact or treatment. Some states extend this to seven years. Check your state board.

Controlled substance logs

Two years minimum under federal law; longer in many states. Apply the longer requirement.

Rabies vaccination records

Retained permanently in most states, given their legal significance in bite cases and interstate travel documentation.

Surgical and anesthesia records

Treat as general patient records at minimum. Given their role in malpractice proceedings, longer retention is prudent.

Minor patients

Some states require retention until the patient would have reached a specific age. Verify with your state board.

When in doubt, retain longer. Storage is inexpensive. Defending a records gap is not.

Record Release and Confidentiality

Client records belong to the practice. Clients are entitled to copies of their pet's medical records upon request. Most states require timely release; some define specific timeframes. Charging a reasonable copying fee is permitted in most states. Withholding records for unpaid balances is prohibited in most states and is a common basis for licensing board complaints.

Confidentiality obligations vary by state. Your state veterinary practice act governs what client and patient information you may share and with whom. The AVMA maintains a state-by-state summary of veterinary record confidentiality laws. Consult it when you receive requests from insurance companies, attorneys, animal control agencies, or other third parties.

AI tools and privacy: any client or patient information entered into a general consumer AI tool is processed on a third-party server. De-identify before you paste. The complete workflow is in Appendix B.

Where AI Helps in Documentation Compliance

Drafting compliance policy documents and SOPs for controlled substance handling, record completion timelines, and record release procedures. Creating staff training materials on logging requirements and what to do when a discrepancy is found. Generating blank controlled substance log templates with all required fields for staff to complete by hand. Producing internal audit preparation checklists. Building SOAP note templates that prompt complete documentation.

Where AI does not belong: actual controlled substance log entries, clinical assessment sections requiring your diagnostic judgment, and any document requiring a verified signature or chain of custody.

Chapter 14
De-identification Workflow

Before any clinical information goes into a general consumer AI tool, it must be de-identified. This appendix gives you a simple, repeatable workflow and a quick-reference card you can keep at your desk.

Why De-identification Matters

When you type or paste information into ChatGPT, Claude, Gemini, or Grok, that text is processed by a third-party server. Depending on the tool's privacy settings, it may also be used to improve future model versions.

Veterinary medicine is not subject to HIPAA, which applies to human healthcare. But your state veterinary practice act almost certainly imposes confidentiality obligations on client and patient information. That professional obligation exists independently of any federal mandate.

De-identification removes the information that would allow a specific client or patient to be identified from the text. It takes ten to fifteen seconds. Once it becomes habit, you won't notice the time it adds.

The Five-Step Workflow

Step 1: Replace the patient name

"Max" becomes "a 7-year-old male neutered Labrador Retriever." Keep the signalment: species, breed, age, sex, reproductive status. Remove the name.

Step 2: Replace the owner name and all contact information

"Mrs. Chen" becomes "the owner." Remove all owner names, addresses, phone numbers, and email addresses.

Step 3: Remove account numbers and financial information

No patient record numbers, invoice numbers, or financial account details belong in a public AI tool.

Step 4: Review for any remaining identifying details

A rare breed in a small community combined with a distinctive presentation might be identifiable even without a name. When in doubt, generalize.

Step 5: Paste the de-identified version

What goes into the AI tool should contain only clinical information: signalment, history, exam findings, diagnostics, and plan. No names, no contact information, no account numbers.

Quick Reference: What Stays and What Goes

Keep in (clinical information)

Species, breed, age, sex, reproductive status. Chief complaint and duration. Owner-reported history in general terms (diet, environment, behavior changes). Examination findings and vital signs. Diagnostic results. Medications administered or dispensed (generic names, doses, routes). Plan and follow-up instructions.

Remove (identifying information)

Client full name, nickname, or initials. Patient name. Client address, city, phone number, email. Account number or invoice number. Any detail that could identify a specific animal or owner in your community.

Edge cases

A highly distinctive case in a small community: generalize the breed or omit contextual details that are not clinically necessary. A patient with a long history: de-identify each element before pasting, or summarize the relevant history in clinical terms rather than copying records verbatim. A case involving a publicly identifiable individual: if the case is identifiable from clinical details alone, do not use a public AI tool for documentation.

Anonymized

Example

Raw notes (not ready for AI tool)

"Max Chen, 7-year-old MN Labrador, Mrs. Chen brought him in for vomiting x3 days. She says he got into the trash four days ago. Eating some, drinking well. No blood in vomit. On exam: mild cranial abdominal pain, otherwise unremarkable. BCS 5/9, temp 102.1, HR 88, RR 24. CBC/chem pending. Started Cerenia 60mg SQ, sent home metronidazole 500mg BID x5 days and bland diet. Recheck if not improving in 48 hours or if vomiting worsens."

De-identified version (ready for AI tool)

"7-year-old male neutered Labrador Retriever, presented for vomiting x3 days following possible dietary indiscretion. Owner reports some food intake, normal water consumption, no hematochezia or hematemesis. Physical exam: mild cranial abdominal pain on deep palpation, otherwise within normal limits. TPR within normal range. CBC/chemistry panel pending. Administered Cerenia 60mg SQ. Dispensed metronidazole 500mg BID x5 days and recommended bland diet. Owner advised to return if not improving in 48 hours or if vomiting worsens."

What changed: patient name removed, owner name removed, replaced with clinical signalment and "the owner" where needed. Everything clinically relevant is preserved.

Print and Post: Quick Card

Before pasting into AI: remove names (patient and owner), remove contact information, remove account numbers. Keep: species, breed, age, sex, history, exam findings, diagnostics, plan. Ten seconds. Every time.

Chapter 15

Recommended Tools and Resources

This appendix provides a current overview of AI tools relevant to veterinary practice, organized by category. The tool landscape changes rapidly. Pricing, features, and availability shift. Verify current details directly with each vendor before making a purchasing decision.

General-Purpose AI Tools

These are the tools covered throughout this book for documentation drafting, client communication, CE preparation, and practice operations. All have free tiers that allow you to start without a subscription.

ChatGPT (OpenAI) | chat.openai.com

Free tier capable for all workflows in this book. Paid tier (ChatGPT Plus, approximately $20/month) provides access to more capable models and higher usage limits. Most widely used general-purpose AI tool. Review OpenAI's privacy settings: the default settings for some account types allow conversation data to be used for model training. Adjust in account settings if this is a concern.

Claude (Anthropic) | claude.ai

Free tier capable with daily usage limits. Paid tier (Claude Pro, approximately $20/month). Particularly strong on natural-sounding prose and following nuanced instructions. Tends toward conservative output on uncertain clinical content. Review current privacy terms at claude.ai.

Gemini (Google) | gemini.google.com

Free tier capable. Paid tiers available through Google One or Google Workspace plans. Integrates directly with Gmail and Google Docs. If your practice runs on Google Workspace, Gemini's integration reduces friction for staff already working in that environment.

Grok (xAI) | x.com

Available through the X platform. Free tier available; bundled with X Premium. Direct, conversational tone. Real-time access to information posted on X. Most suitable as a supplementary tool.

Practical note on tool selection: the prompts in this book work with all four tools. Pick one, use it consistently for the first thirty days, and develop a feel for how it responds before expanding. Consistency builds skill faster than tool-switching.

Veterinary-Specific AI Documentation Tools

This is a distinct and rapidly evolving category. These tools are purpose-built for veterinary documentation, typically using ambient listening to capture exam room conversations and generate SOAP notes automatically. These tools are a different product from general-purpose AI tools. They are more specialized, more expensive, and, for the right practice, significantly more efficient.

Key questions before choosing a veterinary AI scribe

Does it integrate with my PIMS, and how deeply? Read-only pull of patient data and bidirectional write-back are meaningfully different capabilities. Was it trained on veterinary-specific language, or is it a general AI model adapted for veterinary use? Does it support the species and specialties I see? Does it work offline? (Relevant for ambulatory and large animal practitioners.) What are the security certifications? Look for SOC 2 compliance at minimum.

Tools currently in active use as of early 2026. Verify current status, pricing, and features directly with each vendor before committing.

HappyDoc | happydoc.ai

Ambient AI scribe with deep bidirectional PIMS integration for Avimark, Cornerstone, ImproMed, ezyVet, and other major systems. Flat-rate pricing covering unlimited users per clinic. Preferred by practices on legacy PIMS platforms where integration depth matters.

CoVet | co.vet

Ambient AI scribe and clinical documentation tool. Large template library covering general practice, equine, exotics, and emergency. Team-based workflow support allowing technicians and assistants to contribute to documentation. Offline mobile recording available. Per-user pricing. Originally built for Canadian and international markets; used in U.S. practices as well.

ScribbleVet | scribblevet.com

Ambient scribe with Plumb's drug monograph integration and LifeLearn Sofie clinical decision support. Dental charting support. PIMS integration via browser extension. Acquired by Instinct in January 2026.

Scribenote | scribenote.com

Ambient scribe with SOAP, dental, callback, and dictation note types. Free plan available. Accessible pricing. Desktop widget for rapid PIMS transfer. Consistently rated by solo practitioners and small clinics.

VetRec | vetrec.ai

Y Combinator-backed AI scribe focused on voice-to-SOAP note generation. Broad PIMS compatibility claimed. Premium price point.

VetGeni | vetgeni.com

Per-user pricing with SOAP generation, discharge instructions, treatment plans, surgery reports, a 739-drug knowledge base powered by licensed veterinary references, IDEXX Cornerstone integration, and a client-facing portal.

Otto | otto.vet

Standalone AI scribe with flat-rate unlimited-user pricing. Competitive entry price for small practices. Longest free trial period of tools in this category (21 days).

Independent comparison resources: VetSoftwareHub (vetsoftwarehub.co m) provides independent user reviews and rankings across veterinary AI tools. It is the most useful source for unbiased current comparisons.

PIMS-native AI features: Vetspire, Shepherd TranscribeAI, DaySmart Daisy Voice, and Covetrus AI have each introduced built-in AI scribe capabilities. These are convenient but, based on available user data, typically less accurate than purpose-built dedicated tools. Evaluate them the same way you would evaluate a standalone tool: test on real cases, not just vendor demos.

Veterinary AI Diagnostic and Clinical Support Tools

This is a separate and earlier-stage category from documentation tools. These tools assist with diagnostic interpretation rather than documentation. The verification requirements are higher: always treat AI diagnostic output as one input among several, never as a conclusion.

Veterinary AI radiology

Roughly two dozen companies offer AI software for veterinary radiograph review. Some embed directly in digital radiography units and classify images as they are captured. The American College of Veterinary Radiology published a position statement in 2025 establishing guiding principles for ethical development and use. Key vendors include MetronMind (metronmind.com) and Vetology.ai. Most relevant to practices with high imaging volume or without immediate access to specialist radiology consultation.

ImpriMed | imprimedvet.com

AI-driven drug response prediction for canine and feline blood cancers. Uses individualized cell analysis to predict treatment response before it begins. Relevant for practices managing oncology cases.

PetPace | petpace.com

Remote patient monitoring using AI to analyze physiological data from wearable collars. Relevant for practices managing chronic disease or post-operative monitoring remotely.

VetPawer AVA

AI that handles client phone and chat interactions, creates appointments, and proposes prescription refills by integrating directly with practice management systems.

Professional Resources for Staying Current

AVMA AI Resources | avma.org

The AVMA Task Force on Emerging Technologies and Innovation is developing guidance on AI use in veterinary practice. Current guidance, position statements, and task force updates are posted at avma.org. The AVMA also maintains a state-by-state summary of veterinary record confidentiality laws.

AAHA CE on AI | aaha.org

The American Animal Hospital Association has introduced continuing education programming specifically on AI in veterinary medicine. Available through the AAHA professional development platform.

AAVSB AI Guidance | aavsb.org

The American Association of Veterinary State Boards published an AI guidance whitepaper in 2025 addressing regulatory considerations for AI use in veterinary practice.

JAVMA and AJVR

The Journal of the American Veterinary Medical Association and the American Journal of Veterinary Research have published peer-reviewed literature on AI applications, limitations, and ethical considerations. Searching these journals is the most reliable way to stay current on the evidence base.

VetSoftwareHub | vetsoftwarehub.com

Independent user reviews and comparison guides for veterinary AI tools, including AI scribes, practice management software with AI features, and diagnostic tools.

Cornell SAVY | vet.cornell.edu

Cornell's Symposium on Artificial Intelligence in Veterinary Medicine and associated research represent the most rigorous peer-reviewed work on AI applications in the field.

Table C.1: General-Purpose AI Tools for Veterinary Documentation

This table summarizes the four major consumer AI tools covered in this book. Privacy settings and pricing change. Before committing to any tool for clinical work, review current settings directly in the tool and adjust as needed.

Feature	ChatGPT	Claude	Gemini	Grok
Free tier	Yes	Yes	Yes	Yes (via X)
Paid monthly	~$20	~$20	Google One	X Premium
Prose quality	Strong	Very strong	Strong	Variable
Follows nuanced instructions	Good	Very good	Good	Good
Conversations used for training (default)	Yes, adjustable	No by default	Check policy	Check policy
Workspace integration	Third-party	Desktop apps	Deep Google	Limited
Best for	General documentation	Nuanced communication	Google users	Support tasks

Table C.2: Veterinary-Specific AI Scribes

Selected tools in this category. Pricing, features, and availability change. Verify current details directly with each vendor before making a purchase decision.

Tool	Pricing model	PIMS integration	Offline	Species focus
HappyDoc	Flat-rate per clinic	Deep bidirectional	Limited	Small animal, some exotic
CoVet	Per-user	Bidirectional, major PIMS	Mobile	Small animal, equine, exotic
ScribbleVet	Per-user	Browser extension	No	Small animal, dental
Scribenote	Free tier + per-user paid	Desktop widget	No	Small animal
VetRec	Premium per-user	Broad compatibility	No	Small animal
VetGeni	Per-user	IDEXX Cornerstone	No	Small animal
Otto	Flat-rate unlimited	Standalone	No	Small animal

Table C.3: Evaluation Checklist for a Veterinary AI Tool

Before committing to a paid AI tool for your practice, ask the following. Ask in writing. Vendors that cannot answer clearly are vendors to approach cautiously.

1. What species and specialties does this tool support, and has it been vali-

dated for each?

2. What PIMS does it integrate with, and how deep is that integration (read-only, read-write, or full bidirectional)?

3. What happens to my data? Is it retained? For how long? Is it used for model training?

4. Does the vendor offer a business associate agreement or equivalent data-handling contract?

5. What is the tool's security certification status (SOC 2 Type II at minimum for enterprise tools)?

6. What happens when the tool gets something wrong? What is the error rate, and how is it measured?

7. What level of training is provided for my staff, and is there a support channel if we run into problems?

8. What is the cancellation policy? Is there a trial period?

9. Does the tool handle offline situations, if I practice ambulatory or in field conditions?

10. How often is the tool updated, and how are changes communicated to users?

Chapter 16

Your Personal AI Policy Template

Chapter 1 asked you to write down your own AI policy before you started using the techniques in this book. This is the template. Fill it in. It takes fifteen minutes. Keep it somewhere you can find it.

There is no right answer for most of these fields. The goal is to make your decisions explicit before you are in the middle of a busy clinic day. A written policy also gives you a clear, honest answer if a staff member or client ever asks how you use AI in your practice.

Print this page, fill it in by hand, and file it. Or transfer it to a document on your computer. Either way: write it down.

Practice Information

Practice name:
Your name and credentials:
Date written:
Date last reviewed:

Tools I Use

List the specific AI tools you use or plan to use. General-purpose tools (ChatGPT, Claude, Gemini, Grok) and any veterinary-specific tools (ambient scribes, diagnostic tools) should be listed separately.

General-purpose AI tools:

Veterinary-specific AI tools:

What I Use AI For

Check every category that applies to your practice. Add specifics in the space provided.

Drafting SOAP notes for my review:
Discharge instructions and client handouts:
Client communication letters:
Wellness and recall reminders:
Estimate and financial communication:
Staff and operational (SOPs, memos, job postings):
Continuing education preparation and research:
Other uses specific to my practice:

What I Will Never Use AI For

These are your hard limits. The following are a reasonable baseline for any veterinary practice. Add your own in the space provided.

Clinical diagnosis or treatment decisions. Controlled substance log entries. Any document I will not personally review before it leaves the practice. Any input containing client names, patient identifiers, or private information that has not been de-identified.

Additional limits specific to my practice:

De-identification Standard

Before any clinical information goes into a general consumer AI tool, I will remove: client full name, patient name, client contact information, and account or record numbers. The de-identification workflow in Appendix B is my standard.

Any additional de-identification steps specific to my patient population or community:

My Review Process

Every AI-generated document that touches a patient or client will be read in full before I approve it. I will pay specific attention to:

Drug names and spelling. Dosages and routes of administration. Any clinical claim or recommendation. Tone and accuracy of client-facing language. Anything flagged by the AI as uncertain.

Any additional review steps I apply to specific document types:

Staff Use

If staff members in your practice use AI tools, document your expectations here.

Staff members authorized to use AI tools:

Tools they are authorized to use:

Tasks they are authorized to use AI for:

Review and approval process before AI-generated staff work is used:

Client Disclosure

Disclosure norms for AI use in veterinary practice are still evolving. Note your current approach here so it is documented and consistent.

My current disclosure approach when clients ask about AI use in my practice:

Review Schedule

This policy should be reviewed at least once a year, or whenever you adopt a new tool or the professional guidance from the AVMA or your state board changes significantly.

Next scheduled review date:

Fill this in before you go to Chapter 3.

Chapter 17
Glossary

Definitions for terms used throughout this book, written for practicing veterinarians rather than for technologists.

Ambient documentation

A category of AI tools that listen to conversations in the exam room and generate structured clinical notes automatically, without the veterinarian typing or dictating. Also called ambient scribes. The conversation is processed and converted into a SOAP note or other record format, typically within seconds of the appointment ending.

API (Application Programming Interface)

A structured way for one piece of software to communicate with another. When a veterinary-specific AI scribe "integrates with your PIMS," it does so through an API provided by the PIMS vendor. The depth and reliability of that API integration determines how smoothly the two systems work together.

Artificial intelligence (AI)

A broad term for computer systems designed to perform tasks that typically require human intelligence, such as understanding language, recognizing patterns, and generating text. In the context of this book, AI refers specifically to large language models used for text generation and general-purpose chat tools built on them.

Automation bias

The tendency to over-trust or under-scrutinize output produced by an automated system. In a clinical context, automation bias is the risk that a veterinarian accepts AI-generated documentation without adequate review because the output looks authoritative and professionally formatted. Recognizing this tendency is the first step to counteracting it.

BAA (Business Associate Agreement)

A contract that governs how a third-party service handles protected information on behalf of a healthcare provider. BAAs are a requirement under HIPAA for human healthcare. Veterinary medicine is not subject to HIPAA, but some veterinary-specific AI tools offer BAA-equivalent contracts that specify data handling obligations. If you are evaluating an enterprise AI tool for your practice, the data-handling contract is worth reading before signing.

Context block

A paragraph of background information provided at the start of a prompt to orient the AI tool. A species-specific context block for an exotic patient, for example, might include the species' physiological characteristics, common drug sensitivities, and known gaps in AI training data. Context blocks improve output quality by reducing the degree to which the tool must rely on general assumptions.

Context window

The amount of text an AI model can consider at one time, measured in tokens. A model with a small context window will lose track of information from earlier in a long conversation. Modern consumer AI tools have context windows large enough for most veterinary documentation tasks, but if you find the tool losing track of earlier instructions in a long session, starting a new conversation often helps.

Controlled substance log

The required record of every dispensing or administration event involving a Schedule II through V controlled substance in a DEA-registered veterinary practice. Federal law requires these logs to be maintained separately by schedule, with specific fields per entry, and retained for a minimum of two years. State requirements may be more stringent. AI has no role in the actual log entries.

Data retention

The length of time a tool keeps your data after you use it. Different AI tools have different retention policies, and some distinguish between data kept for service improvement (which is retained longer) and data kept only for operational purposes (which is deleted sooner). For a practicing veterinarian, the most important retention questions are: does this tool retain my conversations, and if so, for how long, and who can access them.

De-identification

The process of removing information that could identify a specific client or patient before entering clinical text into a general-purpose AI tool. De-identified text retains clinical content (signalment, history, exam findings, diagnostics, plan) while removing names, contact information, and account numbers. The complete workflow is in Appendix B.

DEA (Drug Enforcement Administration)

The federal agency that regulates controlled substances in the United States under the Controlled Substances Act. Veterinary practices that dispense or administer controlled substances must hold a DEA registration and comply with federal record-keeping requirements, including controlled substance logs.

Embedding

A numerical representation of a piece of text that an AI model uses internally to understand meaning. You'll rarely interact with embeddings directly as a veterinary user, but the term appears in technical documentation of AI tools. When a vendor describes a tool as using "semantic search" or "vector search," it is using embeddings under the hood.

Few-shot prompting

A prompting technique where you give the AI tool two or three examples of what you want before asking for the final output. "Here are three examples of how I write discharge instructions. Match this style in the instruction I'm about to ask you to write." The examples dramatically improve the output quality.

Fine-tuning

The process of additional training on a specialized dataset to make a general AI model better at a specific task. Some veterinary-specific AI scribes are fine-tuned on veterinary clinical text, which is why they handle species-specific terminology better than general-purpose tools. Fine-tuning is a technical process performed by the vendor, not by the end user.

Generative AI

AI systems that produce new content, such as text, images, or audio, rather than simply classifying or analyzing existing content. The general-purpose chat tools in this book (ChatGPT, Claude, Gemini, Grok) are generative AI systems. They produce output by predicting what text is most likely to follow a given prompt, based on patterns learned during training.

Hallucination

The term used in the AI industry for output that is factually incorrect but presented with confidence and apparent authority. AI tools do not know that they are wrong when they hallucinate. Drug names, dosages, clinical claims, and research citations are common hallucination categories in clinical contexts. The review step exists specifically to catch hallucinations before they enter a patient record or client document.

JSON (JavaScript Object Notation)

A structured data format that AI tools can produce when asked. Useful for advanced users who want the output to drop directly into another system. Most practicing veterinarians won't need JSON output, but it appears in the technical documentation of many AI tools.

Large language model (LLM)

The underlying technology that powers the general-purpose AI tools in this book. A large language model is trained on enormous amounts of text and learns to predict what words are likely to follow other words. This makes LLMs highly capable at generating fluent, contextually appropriate text, and equally capable of generating fluent, contextually appropriate text that is factually wrong.

Latency

The delay between sending a prompt and receiving a response. High latency makes the tool feel slow. Factors include server load, prompt complexity, and the tool's current infrastructure. If you consistently experience latency during your clinical workday, switching to the paid tier usually helps.

Markdown

A lightweight text formatting language that many AI tools use by default. Asterisks become bold, number signs become headings. If you paste AI output into a word processor and it looks strangely formatted, the tool probably produced markdown. You can ask for plain text output instead.

Model drift

The gradual change in an AI model's behavior over time, sometimes following updates by the vendor. A prompt that worked well six months ago may give slightly different output today. Not usually a significant issue for veterinary documentation workflows, but worth knowing about if you notice your saved prompts working less well than they used to.

PII (Personally Identifiable Information)

Any data that can identify a specific individual. In veterinary contexts, PII includes client names, contact information, addresses, and account numbers. Removing PII is the core of de-identification.

PIMS (Practice Information Management System)

The software platform that manages patient records, scheduling, billing, inventory, and other practice operations. Common examples include Avimark, Cornerstone, ezyVet, Vetspire, Shepherd, and Covetrus Pulse. Many veterinary-specific AI scribes integrate directly with PIMS platforms to reduce or eliminate manual copy-pasting of generated notes.

Prompt

The text you type into an AI tool to request a response. In the context of documentation, a prompt is the instruction plus the clinical information you provide. Prompt quality directly affects output quality: specific, well-structured prompts consistently produce better first drafts than vague ones. Chapter 3 covers prompting basics; Chapter 11 is a complete prompt library.

Prompt injection

A security concern in AI tools where an attacker embeds instructions in text that the AI tool processes. Relevant mainly to AI tools that read emails, documents, or external web content on your behalf. Less relevant to ordinary chat-based AI use in a clinical setting, but the term appears in discussions of AI tool security.

RACE (Registry of Approved Continuing Education)

The program administered by the American Association of Veterinary State Boards (AAVSB) that sets uniform standards for veterinary continuing education. Most state veterinary boards accept RACE-approved CE toward license renewal. Veterinarians typically need 20 to 30 CE hours per two-year renewal cycle, depending on their state.

RAG (Retrieval-Augmented Generation)

A technique where an AI tool pulls in specific documents or data at the time of your query to ground its response in reliable information. Some veterinary-specific AI tools use RAG to reference current drug formularies or clinical guidelines when generating output. If you see a tool advertise "connected to the latest AVMA guidelines" or "references Plumb's drug monographs," it's using RAG.

Rate limiting

A restriction on how many times you can use a tool in a given period. Free tiers of AI tools often have rate limits that are hit during periods of heavy use. Paid tiers typically have higher limits.

Signalment

The basic identifying clinical descriptors of a patient: species, breed, age, sex, and reproductive status (intact or altered). Signalment is the information that stays in your text when you de-identify clinical notes. It's the clinical anchor for any AI-generated document and must be accurate.

SOAP note

The standard format for veterinary clinical documentation. SOAP stands for Subjective (owner-reported history and chief complaint), Objective (physical examination findings, vital signs, diagnostic results), Assessment (working diagnosis or differential list), and Plan (medications, diagnostics ordered, follow-up, client instructions). SOAP notes are the primary documentation product in most small animal practices and the highest-return application of AI-assisted documentation in this book.

Structured output

AI output produced in a specific, predictable format (typically JSON or a standard template). Useful for tools that integrate directly with your PIMS. If you are writing advanced prompts, asking for structured output can make the result easier to use downstream.

System prompt

An instruction given to an AI tool that applies to the entire conversation, as opposed to a single message. When you start a prompt with "You are helping a veterinarian draft a clinical SOAP note," you are setting a mini-system-prompt. Some AI tools let you save a persistent system prompt that applies automatically to every conversation; this is useful for practicing clinicians who want consistent tone and constraints applied by default.

Token

The unit in which AI models count input and output. Roughly, one token is equivalent to three-quarters of a word. Usage limits and context windows are typically measured in tokens. For practical purposes, most veterinary documentation tasks use well under a thousand tokens per request.

Training cutoff

The date after which new information was not incorporated into an AI model's training data. Events, research findings, drug approvals, and guideline updates that occurred after the training cutoff are unknown to the model. Always treat AI output on recent or rapidly evolving topics with extra scrutiny and verify against current primary sources.

Training data

The body of text on which an AI model was trained. The quality, breadth, and composition of training data shapes what the model knows, how it communicates, and where its blind spots are. General-purpose AI tools are trained on broad text from the internet and other sources. Veterinary-specific AI scribes are typically trained on or fine-tuned with veterinary clinical text, which improves performance on species-specific terminology, drug names, and clinical documentation patterns.

VCPR (Veterinarian-Client-Patient Relationship)

The legally defined relationship that must exist before a veterinarian can diagnose, treat, or prescribe for a patient. The AVMA model definition requires that the veterinarian has sufficient knowledge of the animal to form at least a preliminary diagnosis, has recently examined the animal or made medically appropriate visits to the premises, and is available for follow-up care. The VCPR belongs to the licensed veterinarian and cannot be held or substituted by any AI tool.

Zero-shot prompting

A prompt given without examples. "Write a SOAP note for the following case" is a zero-shot prompt. For simple tasks, zero-shot works fine. For tasks requiring specific style, tone, or structure, adding examples (few-shot prompting) produces significantly better results.

Chapter 18
A Final Word

A Final Word

Veterinary medicine is one of the harder things a person can choose to do. The training is long and expensive. The emotional weight of the work is real. The administrative burden has grown faster than anyone planned for, and it's taking a toll on practitioners who went into this field to help animals, not to spend evenings finishing charts.

AI won't fix all of that. But it can give some of the time back. Not the time spent in the exam room, not the time spent in surgery, not the time spent having the hard conversations with clients about what their animal is facing. That time is yours and it should stay yours. But the time spent turning your clinical thinking into finished documents: that time can be compressed significantly, and this book has shown you how.

The tools in this book are available to you today, at no cost, without waiting for system integration or vendor contracts or practice management approval. You can open an account, paste in a de-identified set of SOAP notes, and have a draft in thirty seconds. The only thing between you and that first hour of time saved is deciding to start.

Use what you learned here carefully. Review everything. Verify drug names and doses. Keep the clinical judgment where it belongs: with you. The tools are good at drafting. You're the one who knows the patient.

And when you've got a working system and a library of prompts and templates that fit your practice, remember that other veterinarians are still where you were before you read this book. The profession benefits when practitioners share what works. You don't have to teach a seminar. A five-minute conversation with a colleague, a post in a professional group, a mention at the next staff meeting, is enough.

The paperwork was never the point. You knew that on the first day of veterinary school, and you know it now. This book is about clearing it out of the way so you can spend more time on the work that's important.

Made in United States
North Haven, CT
04 November 2026

21760247R00095